THE NEW BLUEPRINT FOR FITNESS™

Mud Run Edition

10 Power Habits for Transforming Your Body

ROGER D. SMITH, PHD

Modelbenders Press

PRINTED IN THE UNITED STATES OF AMERICA

Visit our web site at www.modelbenders.com

Designed by Adina Cucicov at Flamingo Designs
Cover images: © *Selestron76* | *Dreamstime.com*
                     © *Yuri_Arcurs* | *istockphoto.com*

The Library of Congress has cataloged the paperback edition as follows:

Smith, Roger D.
    The New Blueprint for Fitness—Mud Run Edition: 10 Power Habits
    for Transforming Your Body
    / Roger D. Smith.—1ˢᵗ ed.
    1. Health & Fitness: Nutrition, 2. Exercise, 3. Weight Loss
    I. Roger D. Smith II. Title

ISBN 978-1-938590-02-3

TALK TO YOUR PHYSICIAN

This book is a reference volume only, not a medical manual. The information given here is designed to help you make informed decisions about your health. It is not a substitute for any treatment that may have been prescribed by your doctor. If you suspect that you have a medical problem, we urge you to seek competent medical help.

All forms of exercise pose some inherent risks. The author and publisher advise readers to take full responsibility for their safety and to know their limits. The exercises and dietary practices in this book may not be appropriate for you based on your physical condition. They are not a substitute for a regimen prescribed by your physician. As with all exercise and dietary programs, you should get your doctor's approval before beginning. You should present this program to your doctor for advice on following or modifying the program to fit your condition.

Also by Roger Smith

Innovation for Innovators:
Leadership in a Changing World

Advice: Written on the Back of a Business Card

Patterns of Strength! New Habits of Personality,
Intelligence, and Relationships

Becoming the Millionaire Employee

Fortune Cookies:
Small Secrets on How to Make a Fortune

To my first physical trainer, the man who got down on the floor to show a pair of boys how to do pushups, situps, and squats. To the man who took me to buy my first set of barbell weights and went back a year later for more. This book is dedicated to my father, Thomas Lee Smith, for the love that he showed but could not speak.

TABLE OF CONTENTS

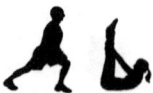

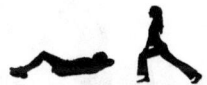

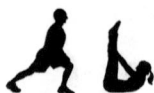

MUD RUN FOREWORD

I had been living the New Blueprint for Fitness for two years when Julie invited me to join a mud run that her fiancé was organizing. She described obstacles like mud pits, wall climbs, floating bridges, and running through rivers. It sounded like the perfect mixture of camping and a playground—as well as a major challenge to my new level of fitness.

When I showed up, the event looked like Mardi Gras in a farmer's field. The "runners" were dressed in everything from Olympic competition gear to superhero costumes and tutu's. The normally sleepy cow pasture was alive with energy, anticipation, fear, and excitement. I had run in many 10K fun runs, but they were nothing like this. At those events everyone was serious about finishing in a decent time and all were dressed like serious runners. Mud Running turned out to be something completely different.

As I inspected some of the obstacles I found earlier waves of runners wading through a shallow river, scaling simple walls, and clambering over stacks of hay bales. But the grand obstacle that was defeating even the best of them was The Gauntlet. This contraption began as an inverted staircase which had to be climbed with your hands. Then everyone shifted to a long set of parallel monkey bars, followed by rings hanging from chains. As I watched the first competitive wave of super-fit athletes work their way through, there were some clever and innovative moves to conquer the obstacle. Many of the women hooked both their feet and their hands around the monkey bars to distribute their weight, one even managed to camber above the bars and crawl across the top. But in spite of fitness, determination, and ingenuity, The Gauntlet took its toll. One quarter of them dropped five feet into the water trap as they transitioned to the monkey bars. Another quarter lost their wet grip in the monkey bars. The next quarter could not manage the grip strength and coordination to traverse the rings. And only one out of four made it across successfully. Though frustrated, everyone took their failure with excitement, climbed out of the water trap and ran off to the next challenge.

When my wave was ready to run, I lined up with a group of girls wearing tutu's with their underwear outside of turquoise leggings, a man in a huge mullet wig, and my buddy who was dressed as Richard Simmons. At the sound of the air horn we all started off to discover what awaited us deep in the woods along this three mile course.

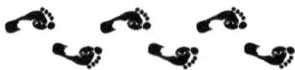

Hog Wild Mud Run turned out to be one of the most challenging, exciting, and fun events I had tried since childhood. Now I understood why these runs were springing up all across the country and attracting thousands of competitors at all fitness levels. I also had a new reason to maintain my New Blueprint for Fitness routine. Some of the obstacles, like The Gauntlet, were beyond my abilities. I ended up in the water trap like almost everyone in my wave. Not only could I enjoy the daily intensity of a workout and the satisfaction of vigorous health, but now I could be invigorated by a weekend test of fitness while wallowing in a mud hole and running through beautiful pastures and woods.

Mud Running will bring out the physical and mental competitor in your personality. It will also return you to a childhood of playing outdoors in touch with nature and all the other children who are as enthused as you are.

A good mud run is now my measure of a good weekend. I have run excitedly through:

- *Savage Race* laid out on the site of a high-end horse steeplechase course, with some of the most difficult obstacles in the country.
- *Superhero Challenge* for aspiring heroes who can go the distance and endure everything thrown at them.
- *Monster Challenge* a great race through the Florida woods and swamps.

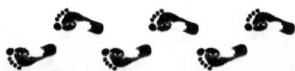

- *Hog Wild Mud Run* circling through Florida farmland, ponds, rivers, and bogs.
- *Mud Endeavor* crisscrossing a motocross valley filled with of obstacles.
- *Tampa Mud Race* circling a local motor speedway sprinkled with new challenges.
- *Prison Break Mud Run* running from snipers with paintball guns.
- And many more ...

Every weekend offers a quest to a new location that I would never see from my office windows, along with a surprising set of physical challenges.

DISCONNECT

In addition to the physical challenge, beautiful scenery, and party atmosphere, these runs give you a chance to disconnect from your daily responsibilities. There are no computers or cell phones on the course. Your electronics will not survive a dip in a river or a slip into a mud pile. You simply have to let go of those connections and get back to living a physical life with other people.

This temporary reprieve may be torture for some, but it can also be as exciting a reason to run as the obstacles themselves. For an hour or two you really cannot be reached and you cannot think about what someone at the end of a digital connection needs from you. It is time for a more primal and natural experience.

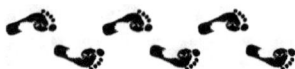

Mud Run Blueprint

The New Blueprint for Fitness is a tool for improving your civilized life—lower fat content, better cardio, stronger muscles, and fewer body ailments. The *Mud Run Edition* adds training and preparation tips to put that fitness to the test. These runs will tax your body's strength, cardio, flexibility, stamina, and full-body performance. The Blueprint was designed to give you all of these. The exercises, nutrition, and rest are not just important parts of a longer life, but also essential for the thrilling events that will occupy your weekends.

Welcome to your *New Run Blueprint for Fitness—Mud Run Edition.*

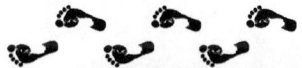

RESTART

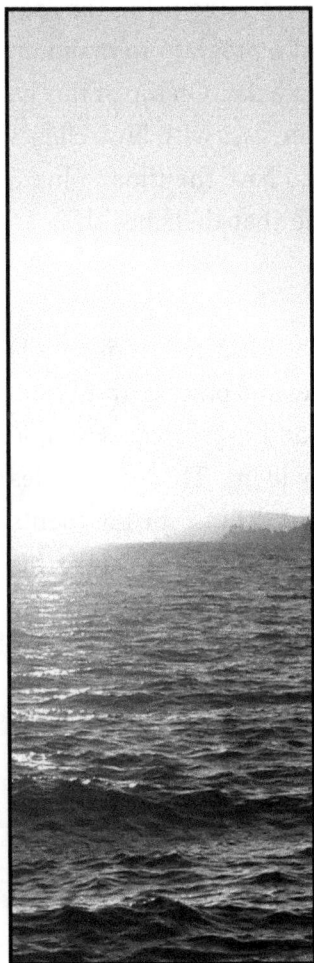

This book presents a New Blueprint for Fitness™ based on the latest discoveries in scientific exercise and nutrition. It was born from my personal experience of abandoning an old blueprint that I had been following for 20 years and adopting a new blueprint as prescribed by expert personal trainers. I began this journey believing that I was in excellent physical condition. But, I was relying on the same exercise and nutrition plan that I had been using for 20 years—my old blueprint. I had put this blueprint together during my high school, college, and young adult years. I was completely unaware that a revolution had taken place in exercise and fitness while I was busy building a career and raising a family.

1

Then Tom showed up.

Tom was a college friend who had spent 20 years building a successful fitness business. He was in better physical condition at age 50 than he had been thirty years before. Tom had studied sports fitness and nutrition and applied all that he had learned to his own health. Over the years, as science discovered and created better ways to remain fit, Tom adopted these discoveries and created a program to maintain ultimate fitness by investing an hour a day. On top of this he created a philosophy of living that he uses with busy clients to convince them that they really do have the time to live a healthy life, as long as they believe that their health is an important priority.

The health and fitness program that I learned from Tom is laid out in this book. Tom's principles and practices are clearly presented, easy to understand, and expressed as simple non-negotiable new habits for daily living. These principles have worked for Tom's own personal fitness, for his clients who have followed them, and for me when I accepted his program as a new blueprint for fitness that was significantly different from what I had pieced together on my own.

I had been using an old and outdated blueprint for fitness for two decades. The results that I achieved were very limited and my internal and external body looked like a middle aged person from the 1970's, which is far from the superior fitness that can be developed using the new scientific knowledge that has emerged in recent years. This science makes up the

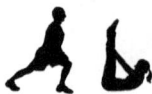

new blueprint that mature people are using to create incredible health and an incredible body.

Tom says ...

— — —

"I believe in the power of an F5 tornado—the Fit 50 year old.

F5 is a mature and powerful adult with a mission to transform their life and their body. In meteorology it is also a storm with wind speeds that can destroy homes and throw automobiles like they are baseballs. Same power."

— — —

THE OLD BLUEPRINT

When we talk about a Blueprint for Fitness we mean the pattern of beliefs and behaviors that people put together to guide their healthy and unhealthy lifestyles. Most people create their own blueprint from physical education classes during high school and college; add the knowledge imparted by their sports coaches; and pickup odd bits of information from magazines and television programs over the years. By the time they reach mature adulthood they have a mind full of confusing facts about health and fitness which they try to apply haphazardly every day. By age 40 most people assume that they have learned everything they need to know about fitness and they stop searching for new tips, tricks, and programs. But the science of fitness marches on without them.

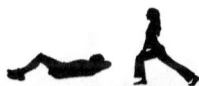

They become stuck to an old blueprint while the leaders in health and fitness are creating a new and more effective blueprint.

This book is a call for you to abandon your old blueprint and adopt a new one which will lead to a level of health and fitness that is far beyond what you have experienced before and beyond what you thought you could achieve at this stage in your life.

Unfortunately, 90% of the population spends 90% of their life ignoring their personal fitness. Every New Year's Day they make a resolution to return to a healthier lifestyle. To accomplish this they brush off their old blueprint for fitness and try to follow it ... for 3 or 4 weeks. This is the time of year when most gym memberships and exercise equipment are sold. The entire nation refocuses on fitness, exercise, and healthy eating for about four weeks. But by the time the calendar clicks over to February, everyone has dropped their New Year's Resolution and is back to their old lifestyle. The gym membership card disappears on the top of the dresser. The new equipment becomes a clothing rack. Television time replaces the daily trip to the gym. The vegetables rot in the refrigerator while the chips and cookies come back into the pantry.

Then there is a second, but smaller, wave of fitness a few months later. These same people return to their fitness resolution around the beginning of May when they think about summer at the beach or pool. They look at their belly and decide they need to get into "bikini shape" before summer

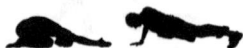

kicks off. So they hunt up that gym membership card, clean the clothes off of the tread mill in the bedroom, and buy a new batch of vegetables. This push lasts 3 to 4 weeks, just like the first one, before they give up, accept their stomach, and purchase a water shirt to cover that bulging belly through the summer.

All of these activities represent the fragmented pieces of an old blueprint for fitness. It does not work well for most of us. A really good blueprint would include exercise, nutrition, and recovery behaviors that are supportive of each other. Everyone needs a blueprint that creates energy and generates a feeling of vibrant health during those first few weeks of enthusiasm. If you are not convinced to change your lifestyle in those critical weeks, then you are not going to stick with your fitness plan.

What does one of these old blueprints look like?

Everyone creates something slightly unique. The dominant characteristic is that it replaces something easy with something hard. Fast food is replaced with homemade salads. Time in front of the television is replaced with time in the gym. In general, these lead to expending more energy, becoming exhausted and wondering when the "energy fairy" will show up to give you the boost you need to keep going.

Here are two of the old blueprints that I used to follow. In general they look pretty good. But the results they deliver are mediocre.

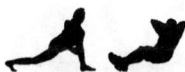

Old Blueprint #1—Muscles	Old Blueprint #2—Cardio
3 workouts per week	Long slow cardio for 60
Rest a day between workouts	minutes
Lift heavy weights	Rest a day between workouts
Use low reps	Conserve energy to reach the
Keep a slow pace to conserve	end of the run
energy	Stretch before the workout
Isolate each muscle	Eat low fat foods
Work for larger muscles	Use carbs like spaghetti and
Stretching is for wimps	potatoes to recover
Cardio is a separate workout	Eat 3 big meals per day
Eat meat and potatoes	
Eat 3 big healthy meals per day	

The muscle blueprint focused on slow weight lifting with plenty of rest between sets and between workout days. The goal was to build muscle mass and conserve energy so I could lift heavier weights. This is a typical pattern created by young men when they are in their early 20's. But, this blueprint is very outdated by the time men reach their 40's, 50's, or 60's. Lifting heavy weights at that age is a certain recipe for injury.

The cardio blueprint is focused on losing weight and building a stronger heart. It is most common among women and overweight people who are worried about a heart attack. Until recently, women did not want to develop muscles, so they targeted a thin frame with solid tone through the use of long cardio workouts. Overweight people are also attracted to this workout because it is easy to begin. It allows them to walk slowly and just keep it up for a long time. But this blueprint

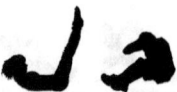

suffers from being too long, too boring, and not addressing the entire body.

THE NEW BLUEPRINT

I was very consistent with the old muscle blueprint for twenty years. But it was dull, routine, and difficult to push to higher levels of fitness, especially as my muscles and tendons became older. What I needed was a new blueprint that incorporated the new science of fitness that had had been discovered in the last ten years and that was appropriate for my more mature age.

A blueprint for fitness at a mature age needs to focus on cardio vascular health, overall muscle balance, protecting the joints and tendons, and feeding the body big doses of nutritious foods. In a nutshell, that blueprint needs to look something like this.

New Blueprint

Six to seven workouts per week
Alternating workout styles
Medium weights and reps
Rapid pace with little rest
Cardio and muscle building together
Compound exercises to work multiple muscles simultaneously
Stretch with every workout
Cardio every day
Fruits or vegetables with every meal
Create a lean body

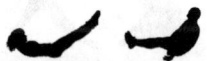

The New Blueprint for Fitness™ organizes the ten most important behaviors and habits that accomplish this so they are supportive of each other. Exercise builds strength, flexibility, and cardiovascular health. This is supported by good nutrition and eating habits. And you learn to rest and recharge throughout the day.

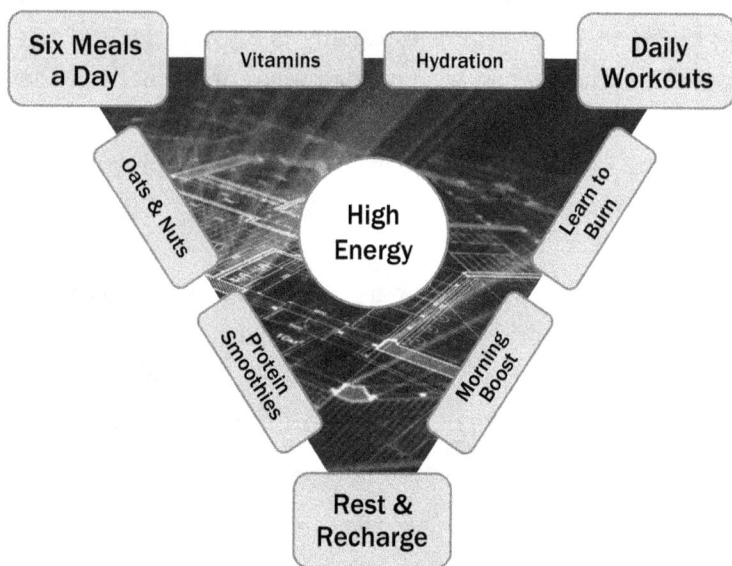

The daily workout program includes four important characteristics

Build strong muscles
    Burn fat
        Breathe your heart into shape
            Bend your joints for flexibility

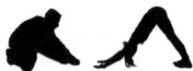

The eating plan calls for fueling the body throughout the day, providing natural foods that have high nutrition and rich flavors. The new blueprint is not just about what you do in the gym every day, but about how you fuel your body so it is able to sustain these workouts and still have energy for your daily activities. That requires a diet full of

Vitamins
Water
Carbs
Protein
Fiber

You will learn more about all of these throughout this book.

FAT AMERICA

The 21st century has given us the highest standard of living and the greatest relief from disease that the world has ever seen. But, this success has also created a massive fitness and weight problem. Millions of people are able to earn enough money to eat all they want and to do as little physical work as possible ... which is exactly what they choose to do. As a result, according to the US Center for Disease Control (CDC), we have a population in which 68% of the people are overweight and underfit, with half of those at a level that is considered obese and physically crippled. That means that the population of the entire country is divided into three pieces—one third is obese, one third is overweight, and one third is at a healthy weight.

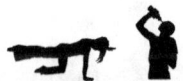

Population Weight Distribution

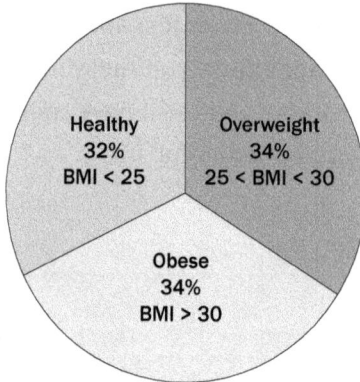

But even those who are considered healthy by this CDC measure often carry a "fat tire" of 10 to 20 pounds around their waist. Few of them exercise regularly. Most have a diet that is too high in animal fats and too low in fruits and vegetables. So even though they are not caught in the CDC's "fat net" they are far from being considered fit, healthy, and prepared for a long and vigorous life.

Our modern lifestyle has created a crisis in which many people face a shorter life expectancy than their parents did. This crisis worries our government leaders because it is contributing to lower job productivity due to health-related absence, early retirement for health reasons, and a heavier burden on the medical care system which is largely supported by federal funds. It also shows up in the ability of the military to enlist and train soldiers. Almost 20% of the teenagers who show up at a military recruiter are already obese. They are in such poor shape that even the military has to turn them down for service.

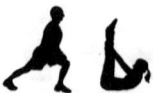

When your body is fat and out of shape, it impacts every-thing else that you do. When that happens to a majority of the population of a country, it impacts the wealth and op-portunity for growth in the entire country.

"Fat America" is a national crisis. Our people work too slowly to compete with the rest of the world and we spend too much of our national wealth on healthcare for a population that is killing itself with excessive food and idleness.

ANOTHER FITNESS PLAN

There are already hundreds of fitness and nutrition books on the shelf, so why should I write and why should you read another one?

I have read many of the books already on the shelf and find that they are filled with excellent information ... usually over-filled with it ... so that the reader comes away more confused than motivated. Those books often include many chapters with photos of exercises, long sections on the chemical activi-ties inside the body, extensive lists of studies that have been done on individual vitamins, and a cookbook full of recipes for healthy food preparation. All of this information is interesting and can be valuable. It is essential for personal trainers who need to coach clients. But the average person is soon lost in all of the details and it does not create a working prescription that they can follow right now to improve their fitness.

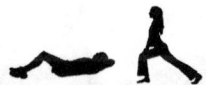

This book is a blueprint. It describes the basic guidelines that you need to build a stronger, leaner, healthier body. That blueprint is crystal clear and laid out so you can work it into your daily life. The ten core behaviors presented here will improve your cardiovascular health, build muscle, improve your digestion, reduce fat, and lead to a longer happier life. This is a New Blueprint for Fitness™ that everyone can understand and anyone can implement.

This book is a clear instruction manual that you can use to change your health, your body, and your lifestyle.

THE POWER TO DECIDE

Are you strong or weak? In control or under control?

When you read about the time, energy, and money that are required to get fit, are you one of the millions who will say "I can't do it!", "I don't have the time", "My job takes all of my energy", or "I can't afford it"?

All of these are great excuses, but none of them are good reasons to avoid fitness and to find yourself in an early grave. The fact is that everyone has the time, energy, and money for the things that are important to them. The excuses are just a smoke screen to avoid admitting that, "Fitness is not important to me."

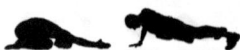

- Who controls your schedule?
- Who controls your energy?
- Who controls your money?

The answer to all of these should be ... you do. You should be exercising the power to decide how you live your own life. Millions of people have given up control of their lives and they wonder why they are not achieving their dreams, they wonder why they are not satisfied. It is because they are working to satisfy someone else's dreams. If you are in this trap, then you may need to read my book *Overcoming the 4 Failures* which will help you to overcome your fear of living your own life.

Take control of your time, your energy, and your money. Invest some of each of these in your own health and fitness. You will be pleasantly surprised that this investment will pay dividends in strength, energy, personal satisfaction, and accomplishment—all within the same 24 hours that you have right now.

Tom says ...

— — —

"1 AM + 1 PM = A Changed Life

Take one fitness action every morning and one every afternoon. Two changes in your entire day are enough to change your fitness, your attitude, your energy, and your life."

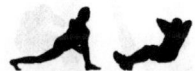

— — —

ONE NEW BEHAVIOR PER WEEK

We are not going to rush into changing everything about the way you live. We are going to take this change one step at a time. The chapters in this book are meant to be read one-per-week.

Read one chapter and put it into practice. At the end of the week you should have gotten into the habit of one new behavior. That is all that we ask of you each week. We are working on a lifestyle change that will stick with you for years. There is no need to rush, become tired, get frustrated, and give up. That will not do you any good at all.

Read one chapter on the first day of your weekend and then purchase the tools that you will need to put that chapter into practice. By Monday morning you should be equipped to practice your new behavior for the rest of the week.

Then move on to the next chapter and repeat the process.

We will start slow and simple, and then build up to more difficult changes. Do not give up. You do have the ability to follow this new blueprint all the way to the end.

Just stick with us and we will all get better together. Hopefully, this book will be your favorite fitness plan. Most people have more than one book on everything that interests them. Cooks have many recipe books. Managers have a library of leadership books. Preachers have a bookcase full of religious

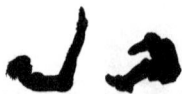

references. Over time you will have the same collection of books, programs, and equipment for fitness. But hopefully, you will point to this book as the one that really got you started with a longterm plan that you could stick with. Hopefully, this New Blueprint for Fitness™ will organize healthy behaviors into a pattern that you start today and continue for the rest of your life.

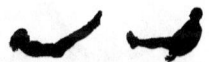

Before you Begin ... Know Your Condition!

This book is a reference volume only, not a medical manual. The information given here is designed to help you make informed decisions about your health. It is not a substitute for any treatment that may have been prescribed by your doctor. If you suspect that you have a medical problem, we urge you to seek competent medical help.

All forms of exercise pose some inherent risks. The author and publisher advise readers to take full responsibility for their safety and to know their limits. The exercises and dietary practices in this book may not be appropriate for you based on your physical condition. They are not a substitute for a regimen prescribed by your physician. As with all exercise and dietary programs, you should get your doctor's approval before beginning. You should present this program to your doctor for advice on following or modifying the program to fit your condition.

Mud Run Disclaimer

Mud Runs and Obstacle events can be challenging athletic events. These also carry the possibility of injury. Every course is different and runners must take caution and make their own decisions about whether an obstacle is safe to attempt. This book does not offer medical or healthcare guidance for these events. Consult a physician or physical training professional for advice on participating in an event in the safest manner possible.

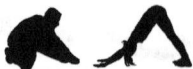

Week 1.
Daily Vitamin

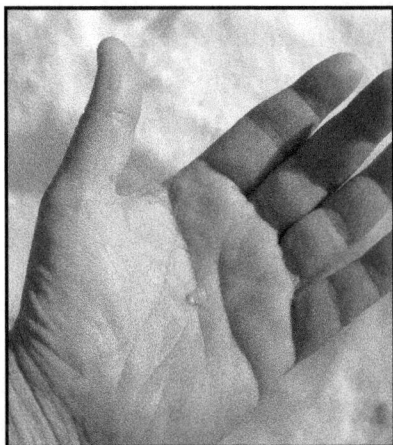

Like a car, your body needs clean fuel and fluids to operate at its best. A car might run fine for years without much maintenance. But inside it is wearing out faster than it should. Without the fresh fluids that reduce friction, your car will wear itself out in half the time that it would if it were well maintained. You can ignore your car's needs and wear it out in 50,000 miles, or you can take care of it and it will keep running for 100,000 miles and more.

Your body is very similar to this. You need nutrients to make everything inside function smoothly for 100 years. If you do not do this, you will wear out around age 50. Most of these essential nutrients are found in the foods you buy at the grocery store. It is generally true that a diet rich in vegetables, fruits, grains, nuts, dairy, and lean meats will deliver all of the nutrients that you need to run your engine for 100 years.

But, be honest, do you really want to eat a spinach and kale for lunch every day to insure that you get the vitamin K that they contain? Do you want to eat carrots every day of your life to get the vitamin A and carotene in them? 99% of the population is just not interested in living in a dietary straight jacket like that.

That is where vitamin and mineral supplements are a big help.

These little pills insure that you get most of the essential vitamins and minerals that you need every single day, not just on the days that you are able to make a special salad, consume a half dozen pieces of fruit, and drink several glasses of milk. They help you enjoy the foods you eat, not become a slave to a regimented menu.

There remains a large and vocal group of health enthusiasts who believe that an all natural diet and lifestyle will create the highest levels of good health and fitness. Their reasoning is that the human body has evolved over millions of years to function in harmony with nature. This is a very seductive and idyllic philosophy. But it is wrong. Left to its natural state, the average body will breakdown and die around age 40.

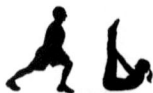

It will suffer from every disease that modern medicine has spent centuries curing and that modern nutrition has been designed to overcome. Just as modern medicine can eliminate disease and help you live longer, modern nutrition and exercise can improve your fitness and health beyond their natural state.

Scientific fitness, nutrition, and health will allow you to live twice as long as "natural man" and do so with much less suffering. New discoveries in food and vitamins are a significant advancement that has led to longer, healthier lives. You should take advantage of these discoveries.

Your first step in the New Blueprint for Fitness™ is to take a multivitamin and mineral tablet every day.

It's that simple. It will add only 30 seconds to your morning routine.

SO MANY CHOICES

Which vitamin product should you use?

There are literally hundreds to choose from. They all seem to be unique and different. But they are not. Most of the differences are just in the packaging and marketing.

Vitamins are made in a small number of pharmacies around the world. Most of the brands that you see on the shelf design their own unique recipes of ingredients and then send those

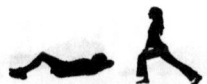

to a commercial pharmacy to be manufactured. The brand on the shelf is a unique combination of contents, shape, color, coating, and printing on the pills, as well as the label, shape, and color of the bottle. But most vitamin tablets are made from very similar ingredients. They are all nearly equal in "quality", a marketing term that is meant to differentiate the expensive products from the inexpensive ones.

If you already have a bottle of vitamins that is not expired, then that is the right one to start taking today.

If you do not have a bottle, then you have many options to choose from on the shelf. You need to find something that is acceptable to your body and your tastes. Look for the following:

Size. The pill should be something that you are comfortable swallowing or chewing every day. The best vitamin is the one that you will actually take, not the one with the best ingredients that will stay in the bottle for years.

Smell. Some vitamins have an odd smell. If that turns your stomach, then choose something else.

Taste. Many people think a vitamin should taste like candy. If that is you, then get a gummy or chewable vitamin that tastes great, or a small tablet that you can't taste at all.

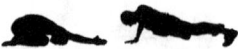

One Daily. Some vitamins are designed to be taken two, three, or six per day. That is too complicated. Choose a vitamin that has everything you need in one single pill.

Cost. We all have financial limits. Choose a vitamin that you can afford to purchase regularly for the rest of your life.

Tom Says ...

— — —

"Visit your local health food or vitamin store to browse the products. Ask the employees for help in finding a vitamin that meets your needs in the size, smell, taste, dosage, and cost categories. They can help you avoid mistakes that will waste your money on a vitamin that you will not use."

— — —

It would be great if a multivitamin tasted like a piece of fruit or candy. But there are so many ingredients packed into such a small tablet that it creates a unique flavor that most people do not like very well. When you put your entire daily supply of ascorbic acid (Vitamin C) into a tiny pill, it is going to taste very sour. When you pack zinc, magnesium, and potassium into a pill there is going to be a metallic taste to that pill. Most people adapt to this taste quickly. But some use gummy vitamins or very small pills for their entire lives so they can avoid this taste. Choose the option that works best for you ... as long as it is not the option of skipping your daily vitamin.

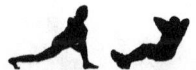

CONTENTS

Even though we recommend that you just pick up a good brand of vitamin at the store, some of you may be interested in what the minimum ingredients should be in a vitamin. Your vitamin should have at least the following Estimated Average Requirements (EAR) established by the United States Institute of Medicine. Since every person has a different body type and metabolism, it is impossible to set a minimum requirement that is optimum for everyone. That is why the Institute of Medicine calls this the "estimated average". This is a good middle-of-the-road recommendation.

Vitamin	EAR
Vitamin A	800 mcg
Vitamin D	5 mcg
Vitamin E	12 mg
Vitamin C	80 mg
Vitamin K	75 mcg
Thiamin	1.1 mg
Riboflavin	1.4 mg
Niacin	16 mg
Vitamin B6	1.4 mg
Folic Acid	200 mcg
Vitamin B12	2.5 mcg
Biotin	50 mcg
Pantothenic Acid	6 mg

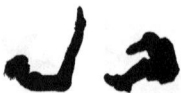

Minerals	EAR
Potassium	2000 mg
Chloride	800 mg
Calcium	800 mg
Phosphorus	700 mg
Iron	14 mg
Magnesium	375 mg
Zinc	10 mg
Copper	1 mg
Manganese	2 mg
Fluoride	3.5 mg
Selenium	55 mcg
Chromium	40 mcg
Molybdenum	50 mcg
Iodine	150 mcg

"mg" is the abbreviation for milligram. "mcg" is a microgram, or 1,000ᵗʰ of a milligram. "IU" is an International Unit, which can be converted into "mg", but the conversion is different for every vitamin.

If you compare these tables to the ingredient lists on even the most economical vitamins you will find that the contents of most brands easily cover all of these, and in most cases go far beyond. The contents of most vitamin pills are driven by research into improving human performance and health, not just remaining alive without a severe vitamin/mineral deficiency. The EAR gives the lowest numbers for preventing diseases like scurvy and rickets.

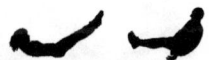

Some of the more unique supplements available in stores are driven by advanced research, folklore, and marketing. In a world where thousands of competitors can create a vitamin tablet that meets the needs of the human body and it can be sold for pennies a day, competitive companies really need some way to differentiate themselves. They do this by remaining plugged into the latest research and creating a vitamin that incorporates new ingredients that have recently been shown to have beneficial results. They also create a unique brand by advertising their tablets as containing more of everything good or of higher "quality" than their competitors.

Eventually you can experiment with these advanced vitamin tablets as much as your wallet will allow. But it is unlikely that you will see or feel any difference from taking any of the good solid, average vitamins on the shelf in every health food store, grocery chain, and discount center. When you are just beginning your vitamin supplement routine you should use any tablet that you like and can afford. Later you will find yourself comparing all of the labels on the shelf in an attempt to get the best ingredients for the money you have to spend.

People with special health situations should consult their physicians about the right type and dosage for their vitamins. This is especially important for women who are pregnant or nursing; as well as those taking medications and anyone who is alcoholic. Some vitamins interact with medications and alcohol in unique ways that require professional medical advice.

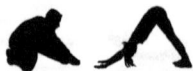

EFFECT

Taking a vitamin/mineral tablet is not like downing an energy drink. You will not feel an immediate rush of energy. Rather, over time, you should notice subtle, but solid, improvements in your health. When your body has these nutrients it can perform its daily activities better. This includes a sound sleep, regular and reliable digestion, preventing and repairing injuries to the joints, stable blood chemistry, and improved oxygen absorption during exercise. To really notice each of these you would need to keep a journal of your habits before taking the vitamins and again for a couple of months after taking them. The changes are subtle, but they are there. It is easy to take these for granted because they are not the same rush that you get from caffeine or sugar.

A multivitamin every day should become a habit like bathing in the morning. It is something that you never forget because it is a necessary step in your morning routine. Buying a vitamin takes an additional 60 seconds at the store. Actually taking the tablet is another 30 seconds per day. There is really no reason that you cannot fit this essential and important new habit into your day.

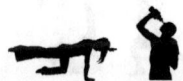

BEYOND THE MULTIVITAMIN

If you talk to health nuts, athletes, and back-to-nature enthusiasts about their vitamin supplements, you will find that all of them take more than just a single multivitamin. They all swear by a different combination of supplements that enhance their specific activities. In most cases, these devotees have built up their stock by reading books and articles or talking to other healthy people that they respect. They have arrived at a mixture that works well for them both physically and psychologically.

If you stick with the New Blueprint for Fitness™ program, you will find yourself on that same journey in a few months or years. But, right now you are just getting started and there is no reason to make this more complicated than it needs to be. Today you need one simple habit that you can continue for the rest of your life. Boosting this to higher levels will come later.

WEEKLY SHOPPING LIST

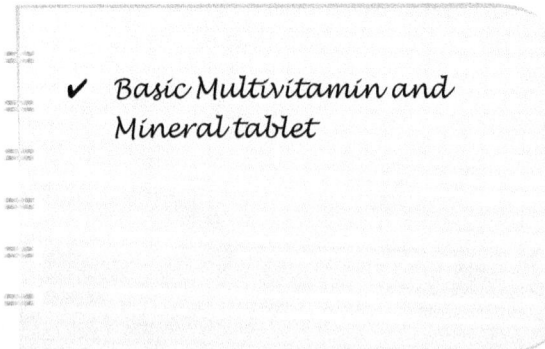

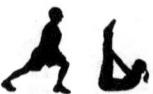

✔ *Basic Multivitamin and Mineral tablet*

Mud 1.
Vital Muderals

Mud runners experience more cuts, scrapes, muscle cramps and pulls than your average fitness enthusiast. In the gym, the sharp edges have been polished off. But when the great outdoors, wooden walls, and metal monkey bars are your gym, you will quickly get a few scuff marks on your frame.

A good daily vitamin is essential to insure that your body is prepared to fight any infections that could come from these minor injuries, as well as the antioxidants that will help you heal and rebuild from an injury.

You will walk off of the obstacle course with a scrape from a tree, a cut from a wooden wall, a poke from a metal brace, or a splinter from a fiberglass boat hull (yes, you will find those on some courses). These are not something to be afraid of. The human body is made to recover and heal itself naturally. Your daily vitamins and minerals will insure that you heal more completely and faster than you would otherwise.

Supplements will also sharpen your mental focus when training and competing. On a mud run course you always need to be looking beyond the immediate obstacle to the landing spot on the other side, insuring that you are ready to dismount gracefully without injury. A good vitamin mix in your brain will help you maintain this focus longer and contribute to fewer injuries.

For the good of your long-term participation and enjoyment in this sport you need to keep the vitamins and mineral levels up and flowing through your body.

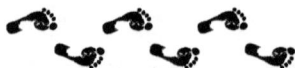

Week 2.
Morning Metabolism Boost

Every night your body and mind go into a short hibernation. The relaxation flows through your arms, legs, back, and mind. It is a cyclical daily recovery ritual.

But everyone knows that the peace and relaxation that come from a night of sleep do not start the minute that you put your head on the pillow. It takes time to transition from your alert, awake, and thinking persona to your relaxed, resting, and sleeping persona.

This same process applies when you wake up in the morning.

When your eyes open, the process of coming fully awake, becoming fully "on" takes some time. You may stand up, but you are not at full speed for several minutes or even an hour. Most people use a shower and a morning coffee to bring their mind and body up to full speed.

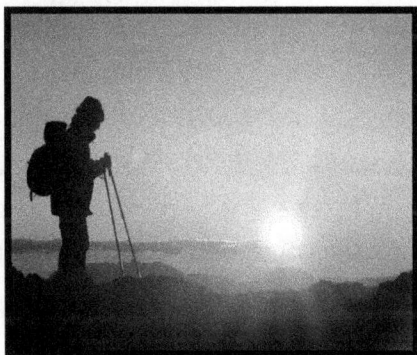

But what about your metabolism?

Your body burns calories at different rates when you work, sleep, and exercise. While sleeping your metabolism has shifted down to its slowest rate for the entire day. The longer that you wait to start your metabolism back up in the morning, the fewer calories that you will burn all day, and the higher your body weight will be. One step in building a lean and healthy body is to fully engage your metabolism as soon as possible. You need a metabolism boost in the morning just like you might need a morning caffeine boost.

If your metabolism remains on "night slow" for just one additional hour of your waking day, then that is a 6% decrease in your daily metabolism. That could mean as much as a 6% increase in your weight. Or a lost opportunity to drop 6% of your body weight with a very small investment in physical activity.

The second behavior that you are going to add is a metabolism boost every morning. You are going to invest 15 minutes each morning to drop 6 to 18 pounds of body fat over the span of a single year.

Tom was brilliant in realizing and explaining how easy it is to get an edge on weight loss and building healthy muscle with a very small investment in jump starting your metabolism the first thing in the morning.

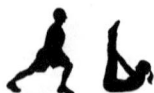

This week you are going to start a new habit of waking up 20 minutes earlier than usual. You are going to make room in your day for a little early morning exercise. This is not a full workout. It is just a jumpstart to get your day going. Most people hate to lose even a few minutes of sleep, but I promise you that this one is going to create more energy than it takes away.

MORNING BOOST

When you step out of bed every morning, step directly into some comfortable clothes that are good for a little activity. The best metabolism boost is simply to go for a walk. If the weather allows, step out your front door and start walking. Just walk around the equivalent of a single city block. Walk for about 15 minutes.

During your walk, look at the sky, breathe the morning air, listen to the birds. Make a connection with the world around you. Soak in the richness of a world that has existed for billions of years. Reach out for some of the peace of this ancient world. Notice how relaxed and in-tune it is. Include some of that peace in your own soul.

In addition to being a spiritual commune with nature, this mild exercise will jumpstart your metabolism for the day. The machinery that converts stored fat and calories into energy and muscle will start working for you immediately.

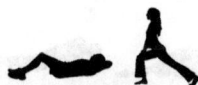

When you return from this little walk around the neighborhood, you are going to finish up with a few calisthenics. These exercises do not require any equipment and can be done in 4 minutes.

TABATA TIME

It is a popular belief that a workout has to be 30 to 60 minutes long to be effective. But, when you use a Tabata circuit you can accomplish a great deal in just 4 minutes.

Dr. Izumi Tabata published a research study in which he showed that, even for conditioned athletes, alternating short periods of intense exercise with short recovery breaks provided more improvements in cardiovascular health than longer periods of exertion at medium levels. This led to the creation of the Tabata workout craze. The simplest of these can be done in just 4 minutes.

4 Minute Tabata Training Set

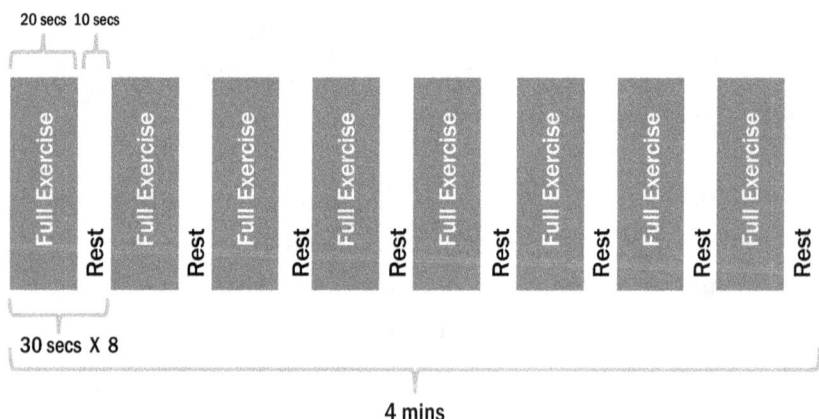

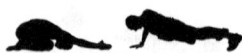

20 secs 10 secs

Full Exercise   Rest   Full Exercise   Rest   Full Exercise   Rest   Full Exercise   Rest   Full Exercise   Rest   Full Exercise   Rest   Full Exercise   Rest   Full Exercise   Rest

30 secs X 8

4 mins

A Tabata Set consists of 20 seconds of exercise, followed by 10 seconds of rest. This short cycle is then repeated eight times. The entire set is finished in just four minutes. A single set is the perfect morning metabolism boost. When you return from your 15 minute walk around the block you are going to pick one of the Tabata sets shown below based on your current fitness level.

Mild	Medium	Hot	Custom
Alternate Toe Touch	Burpee with Jump	Burpee with Push-Up	Create your own combinations.
Jogging in Place	Squat		
Trunk Twists	Push-Up		
Squats	Bicycle Crunches		
Repeat Circuit Twice	Repeat Circuit Twice	Repeat All 8 Sets	

Notice that for the Mild and Medium workouts we have listed 4 different exercises. You go through these in sequence, 20 seconds of the first, 10 seconds rest, 20 seconds of the second, 10 seconds rest, and so on. When you finish all four, go back and do them all a second time.

For the Hot workout we have prescribed one of our favorite exercises—the Burpee with a Pushup. Do this same exercise for 20 seconds of work, 10 seconds of rest, repeated eight times.

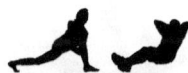

This sounds like a walk in the park. But Dr. Tabata discovered something really powerful. This routine packs a lot of work into a very short period of time. When you finish this your first time you will be impressed.

TABATA TIMER

You can time your Tabata workout by doing the exercise in front of a clock with a second hand. You may also be able to find a programmable timer app for your phone. Or you can buy a special Tabata Timer.

I started by watching the clock for my Tabata circuits. This worked just fine. But I was prone to making mistakes when I was tired. I often forgot which set I was on and sometimes stopped short of the full eight sets.

Tom told me about a fantastic little device called the Gym-Boss® which is a simple timer that can be programmed with alternating exercise/rest intervals. This was the best little device I had ever used to boss me through a Tabata circuit. At $20, it is worth the investment.

After using it for my morning Tabata routine, I even bought a second one to put in my gym bag. I use this one to keep me moving through a weightlifting workout in the gym. It has had a tremendous effect on the intensity of the work that I get done and has significantly shortened my workout times while also making them more intense and effective.

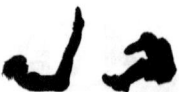

Tom Says ...

— — —

"A 4-minute Tabata workout is the most energizing, healthy, and shortest part of creating a healthy lifestyle. Nothing else can create so much change to your body in just 4 minutes."

— — —

RAINED OUT

Starting every morning with a walk outside is fantastic if you live in California, Florida, or Arizona. But for many locations, the weather is not friendly or cooperative year round. It is also not a safe practice in some cities. If this is the case where you live, then I would recommend using a short indoor workout. You could create this yourself with a couple of Tabata sets. Or you could use one of the many 10 minute workout DVD's. Some of my favorites are:

- Jackie Warner's Power Circuit Training®
- Beachbody 10 Minute Trainer®
- 10 Minute Pilates

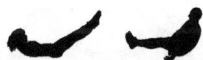

MORNING HUNGER

Once this routine wakes up your metabolism, it will be just a short time before your body realizes that it has not eaten for 8 to 10 hours. When that happens, your brain is going to send a message to your stomach telling it to declare that it is hungry. For some of you this will be a surprising feeling in the morning. If you have conditioned yourself to skipping breakfast or having just a cup of coffee, this sudden need to eat so early in the morning is going to take you back to childhood when your mother forced you to eat breakfast before she would let you leave the house.

This is an excellent change. The purpose of the workout was to switch on your metabolism and becoming hungry is a good sign that you have accomplished this. So, in addition to the benefit of losing a few pounds in the morning, you are going to get back into the habit of having a regular and healthy breakfast.

Most people stop eating in the evening by 8:00pm. If they wake up at 6:00am, then this is a long 10 hour streak without any food at all. If you had gone 10 hours during daylight hours without food you would be ready to chew off your own leg. It would be like eating lunch at noon and not touching food again until 10:00pm. Or like eating a 6:00am breakfast and then working through the entire day without a bite to eat until 4:00pm. This would be a crazy long period without food if you were awake. While you were sleeping, your body was very busy rebuilding your muscles and internal organs.

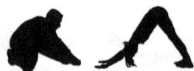

The fuel that you put in at dinner the night before is long gone and there is no fuel left to run your body this morning. But, since you have been sleeping and your metabolism has slowed down, your body and brain have just not realized that they need fuel yet. On top of this hibernation effect, many people use a morning cup of coffee to suppress their appetites. That just makes the nutrition problem worse.

This little workout has awakened your metabolism. Now you have to feed it. Both the metabolism boost and the moderate, healthy breakfast are going to drive your body weight to a new level of fitness.

WEEKLY SHOPPING LIST

✔ GymBoss® Tabata Timer (see Amazon.com, Ebay.com, or Gymboss.com)

✔ Workout DVD (10-15 minute routines)

MUD 2.
MORNING MUDTABOLISM

Mud runs are typically morning events beginning as early as 8:00am and running through the afternoon. That means your body needs to be firing on all cylinders first thing in the morning. A good early morning stretch and flex program is going to get your muscles, joints, metabolism, and mind ready for morning action.

If you typically do your main workout in the afternoon, you also need something short and quick to boost your metabolism in the morning. This is a good time to focus on flexibility, circulation, and your core strength. This is not a second, full out, high intensity event. It is a booster to wake your body up and get you moving for the rest of the day.

As a mud runner, this little workout is also a great time to work on a single focused ability. If you have flexibility problems, then try yoga or Pilates for 10-20 minutes in the morning. If you need more cardio, then try a short, but quick run around the neighborhood. If you are trying to conquer a specific obstacle, then spend 10-20 minutes focused on that specific movement.

Many mud runners need help getting over the eight foot wall, clambering across the monkey bars, or army crawling under barbed wire. Your morning metabolism boost can be a special time to focus on those movements.

Wall Climb. Find a fence or wall in the neighborhood and practice climbing back and forth over the top of it repeatedly. This is a great move for building arm, core, and leg strength. It will help you coordinate all of the muscles that are needed to get over the walls on a course. You will probably not find an eight footer to practice on, but a five or six footer climbed 10 times in a row will be great preparation.

Monkey Bars. There are very few places to find real monkey bars in a neighborhood. If you are lucky enough to live near a school that has a set, then run down there and use them for 10 minutes. Everyone else will have to make do with a doorway chin-up bar. Reach up, bend your knees, and do as many chins as you can. Then hang from the bar while hand walking to different positions on the bar. The newer designs of these bars have multiple hand-holds that can be used this way. The best competitors on the monkey bars traverse them without completely extending their arms. If you have the strength to do this, then you have more control over your arms and body which means you can move faster. It also reduces the amount

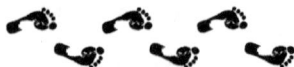

of joint stretch that you will feel after the monkey bars, retaining more strength for other obstacles.

Army Crawl. This is an easy one to practice. Just get down on your stomach and crawl a path through your backyard for 60 seconds. Then standup, stretch, and get down and do it again.

Tabata Obstacles. The Tabata sequence is similar to a mud run course. Though it may seem like an obstacle takes a minute to get through, each one is really just a few seconds of intense work. Then you are up and running to the next one. A Tabata workout will get you used to repeating short bursts of intense work, followed by short rests, then repeated again. The entire four minute workout is a miniature mud run with just eight obstacles on the path.

Running. Workouts in the gym or in your home can stimulate you cardio very effectively. But this is not exactly the same combination of muscles and breathing that is required to actually run 3, 5, or 10 miles in a mud run. If you plan to run the entire course, then you need to run in training as well. A short one mile morning boost is a good beginning.

Once you have tried all of these ideas you should create your own variations.

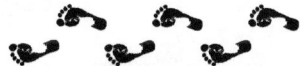

WEEK 3.
OATS & NUTS

Last week we turned on your metabolism the first thing in the morning, which led to a surprising early morning hunger in your stomach. Some of you are out of the habit of eating breakfast so this may have created a problem for you. You need breakfast again for the first time in years and the few options that you remember are not that healthy. In America, there have been three dominant breakfast choices.

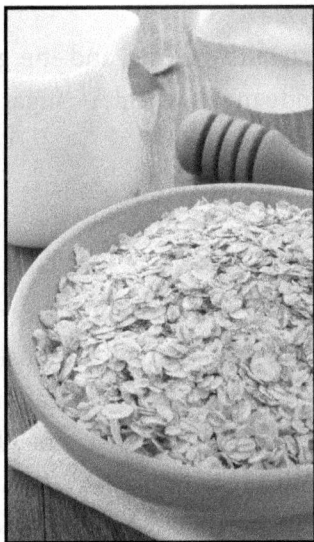

America's Breakfast Habits		
Liquid Breakfast	**Hot Breakfast**	**Cold Breakfast**
Coffee	Fried Eggs	Processed Box
	Fried Bacon	Cereal
	Toast	Milk
	Juice, Milk, or Coffee	

None of these are very good choices. Coffee has no nutritional value at all. The hot breakfast contains too much fat and the cold breakfast contains too much sugar. These bad calories will negate the good work that you have done by waking up your metabolism first thing in the morning. If you are just going to feed on bacon, then it would have been better to let your sleeping metabolism lie rather than to wake it up and make things worse.

Can you imagine a healthy, filling, and energy filled breakfast that does not include meat, wheat, or sugar? Close your eyes and see what comes to mind.

Did you see ... oatmeal?

Oatmeal is an excellent source of complex carbohydrates and fiber for your first meal of the day. Curiously, you do not see many advertisements for simple oatmeal on television. It is so inexpensive and basic that there is not a big profit margin on it like there is on sugar-based cereals. So companies can get a lot more profit for their advertising dollar if they promote something that they made themselves and engineered

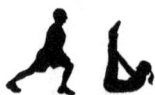

to deliver a unique flavor at very low cost. Oatmeal is just too easy, too natural, and too cheap.

This is going to become one of your new best friends. World-class trainer Jackie Warner says that she uses oatmeal like vitamins. She carries packets with her all the time and cooks one up when she is feeling hungry. The complex carbs, fiber, and water retention of oatmeal will give you fuel, fill your stomach, and avoid the quick blood sugar spike that comes from processed foods. It is one of the few perfect foods.

Oatmeal Nutrition	One Cup
Serving Size	81 g
Calories	307
Total Fat	5 g
Saturated Fat	1 g
Trans Fat	0 g
Cholesterol	0 mg
Sodium	5 mg
Total Carbohydrates	56 g
Dietary Fiber	8 g
Sugars	1 g
Protein	11 g
Vitamins	
Folic Acid	26 mcg
Choline	33 mg
Minerals	
Calcium	42 mg
Iron	3.4 mg
Phosphorus	332 mg
Potassium	293 mg
Selenium	23.4 mcg

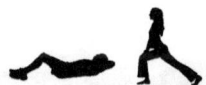

CHOOSING YOUR OATS

You will find dozens of different varieties of oatmeal at the store. These can be divided into two basic categories—those with sugar and those that are plain oats. Guess which one is bad and which one is good?

The flavored varieties with sugar attract children and sugar-addicts. They are easy to sell, can be packaged in any flavor, and have very high profit margins. But, they are not a good choice for healthy living. Skip over every oatmeal package with maple, cinnamon, apples, spices, strawberries, peaches ... and SUGAR. These are designed to attract children and to make everyone fatter.

You need plain oats that you can flavor with healthy ingredients yourself.

In the plain oats category there are three styles—steel cut, rolled, and instant. All of these are made from exactly the same ingredients—plain old oats. The oats are just cut differently to create a different texture.

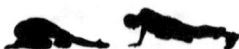

STEEL CUT OATS

Hard-core natural food buffs will insist that nothing beats steel cut oats. A raw handful of this looks and feels like small ball bearings. The original oat nugget is sliced into smaller nuggets with steel blades. The result is a ball or pellet that still has much of the dense fibers that existed in the oat kernel. These dense pieces have a slightly more effective fiber for your digestion. They are also more filling and digest slower because of their density.

But, steel cut oats take 30 minutes to cook up. This does not fit into most people's breakfast and snack schedules. People who are devoted to this form of oats solve this problem by making a big batch on the weekend, and then reheating them for breakfast or a snack throughout the week. Servings can be spooned into a zip-lock bag or plastic container to be taken to work and stored in the refrigerator. When you are ready to eat them, empty into a bowl and pop in the microwave.

Tom Says ...

— — —

"Do not microwave your food in plastic containers. You do not need to digest any more plastic molecules than already slip into your food every day."

— — —

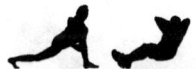

ROLLED OATS

The second best choice is the plain rolled oats, often labeled "Old Fashioned Oats". These are exactly the same oat as in the steel cut box, but instead of slicing the oat nuggets, they have been steamed and run through steel rollers that smash them into flat little oat petals. Rolled oats contain the same fiber and carbohydrates as steel cut oats. But, because they are less dense, they will digest faster in your system. This means that you will probably not feel as full or stay full for as long as with the steel cut oats. But the "complexity" of the carbohydrates has not changed at all. Smashing an oat flat does not turn a complex carb into a simple carb (also known as sugar). This form might contribute a little less digestive assistance than steel cut oats because it digests a little faster. But most people will not notice any difference.

INSTANT OATS

Finally, there are the "Instant Oats". These are exactly the same oats as those in the steel cut and rolled boxes. Instant oats are usually made in the same manner as rolled oats, being smashed into little round petals. But then the petals are cut into pieces so that each is a much smaller piece of the original oat nugget. Because they are smaller, each piece can absorb water faster and it has to absorb less water than the whole rolled oat to be fully cooked. These are instant because the water absorption can happen in as little as 30 seconds in a microwave. So you are less than a minute away from a healthy snack at all times. Also, since the fibers in the oat were both smashed and cut, they are shorter than those in the other two varieties. That means they will provide slightly less help

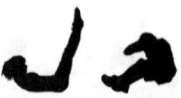

in general digestion. Since these oats digest faster, you will notice that you are not as full nor do you remain full for as long when eating them.

Given three versions of the same basic ingredient, which is the best choice for you?

The answer is easy. The best choice is the one that you will actually prepare and eat every day.

If you have the time and discipline to prepare steel cut oats daily or in a big batch once a week, then do that.

If you can wait for 3 minutes while your oats cook, then use the rolled oats.

If you need to dash into the kitchen and back out with your breakfast, then use the instant oats.

Most people get very motivated to change their diets at the beginning of the year, just before summer, and after reading a book like this. While their enthusiasm is at its highest they set their sights on doing the very best thing that is available—like cooking steel cut oats for 30 minutes every morning. But after the newness wears off, they find that they have chosen the most difficult diet to stick with. So, when their enthusiasm wanes, they drop their new habit entirely rather than adjusting to something that is more practical.

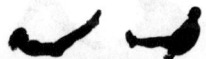

Oats are oats. Just choose the one that you can stick with for an entire year.

BOOSTING THE FLAVOR

I have to admit that oats are very plain tasting. Even the healthiest people give them a little boost. Food companies try to add this boost with a big dose of sugar. They may list the flavor as "Peaches and Crème", but it is really "Sugar and Chemicals". This is a pity because it is so unnecessary. There are healthy, inexpensive, and simple ways to add great flavor to your oatmeal. But you are going to have to do it yourself.

I recommend adding three little ingredients.
1. Start with a small packet of artificial sweetener (Truvia® or Splenda®) to make this simple food a little sweeter.
2. Add some fruit like raisins, cranberry raisins, blueberries, or even a little trail mix.
3. Spice it up with a big shake of cinnamon.

This will create a dish that is far better tasting and much healthier than the sugared versions on the store shelves.

Tom says ...

— — —

"In my desk I have a box of instant oatmeal packets, a bunch of mini raisin boxes, a small shaker of cinnamon, and packets of Truvia®. When I need a snack, I get a coffee cup, pour each of these in and make the best oatmeal in less than 3

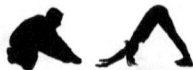

minutes. This will fill you up and keep you away from candy bars all morning."

— — —

AWESOME NUTS

This week you are making two changes to your diet, both of them small.

First—oats. Second—nuts.

Throughout the day you need fuel between your major meals.

Question ... What foods are strong enough to give you energy, build your body, and fill your stomach? At the same time, what is portable, easy to store, and will not spoil?

Answer ... Nuts.

Fruits and vegetables are great and you should not throw them out as snack options. But, most of this country is missing out on one important food in their diets. Nuts and seeds are tiny little packages of protein, carbs, and fats—along with essential fatty acids and micronutrients that your body needs because they come from so few other foods.

Several years ago, there was a fantastic study and a book called *The Blue Zones*. The researchers studied all the longest lived communities on the planet. Each of them had different diets,

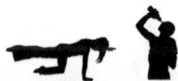

methods for dealing with stress, and routines for physical activity and exercise. But several had one interesting dietary trait in common which was missing from most of our busy lives. They were in the habit of eating nuts regularly. Some were vegetarians who relied on the nuts as a source of protein and fats. But others just used nuts as a snack throughout the day. They reported eating all kinds of nuts—peanuts, cashews, almonds, Brazils, hazelnuts, etc. They enjoyed them raw, roasted, or salted. None of those details mattered. It was only important that nuts and seeds were part of their diet every day.

From a biological perspective, the nut or seed was created with all of the ingredients to launch new life. Everything that a plant needs to get started is encapsulated in the nut. Nuts and seeds are the mother's milk of the plant world. When planted in the ground you just have to add water to unleash the magic that is packaged inside. You should take heed of this power and plant them in your stomach every day. Then add water.

A small, one ounce package of almonds is a great snack. With this tiny package you get 6 grams of protein, the same amount as in a hardboiled egg or a small glass of milk. There are 6 grams of carbohydrates with 3 grams of fiber. The fiber is almost equal to a bowl of oatmeal or a tablespoon of ground flax seed. They contain 14 grams of fat. However, 3 of these grams are polyunsaturated fats which may help reduce cardiovascular disease, and there are 8 grams of monounsaturated fats which may improve your HDL cholesterol.

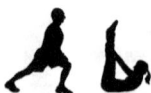

It takes just one seed to grow an entire tree. Each seed or nut is very dense with nutrition so you do not need to eat these by the cup full. Limit yourself to a snack of one or two ounces.

Nut Nutrition	Almonds	Peanuts	Cashews
Serving Size	1 ounce	1 ounce	1 ounce
Calories	161	164	155
Total Fat	14 g	14 g	12 g
Saturated Fat	1 g	2 g	2 g
Trans Fat	0 g	0 g	0 g
Cholesterol	0 mg	0 mg	0 mg
Sodium	0 mg	2 mg	3 mg
Total Carbohydrates	6 g	6 g	9 g
Dietary Fiber	3 g	2 g	1 g
Sugars	1 g	1 g	2 g
Protein	6 g	7 g	5 g
Minerals			
Calcium	42 mg	15.1 mg	12.6 mg
Iron	3.4 mg	0.6 mg	1.7 mg
Phosphorus	332 mg	100 mg	137 mg
Potassium	293 mg	184 mg	158 mg
Selenium	23.4 mcg	2.1 mcg	3.3 mcg

Nuts can be an expensive item. But there are ways around that. First, look for the big canisters at the warehouse stores or grocery stores. You can get all varieties in larger quantities at lower prices. Second, look for individual 1-2 ounce packets that you can store in your desk, auto glove box, or backpack. These give you a single serving that is always handy and usually less expensive than a candy bar.

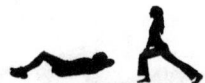

AM AND PM CHANGES

This week you are going to make a hot bowl of oatmeal with dried fruit, artificial sweetener and cinnamon your new breakfast. You will have this at least once a day. Feel free to have another for a morning or afternoon snack if you like.

Then you are going to add nuts to your snacking routine one time during the day. You can choose any nut that you like. It can become your afternoon snack along with a piece of fruit. It can be your post workout or evening snack along with a big glass of water.

WEEKLY SHOPPING LIST

✔ Plain Oatmeal (steel cut, rolled, or instant)

✔ Dried Fruit (raisins, cranberry raisins, blueberries)

✔ Truvia® or Splenda® packets

✔ Bucket of Nuts (almonds, cashews, peanuts, etc.)

✔ Single Serving Packets of Nuts

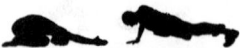

MUD 3.
HORSE AND MONKEY FOOD

The habit of breakfasting on complex carbohydrates and snacking on a natural mixture of nuts is great for maintaining a high energy level throughout the day. Athletes of all types use this strategy to fuel their bodies and it is just as good for a weekend mud runner.

Prior to a race you need fuel that will stick with you until the end of the race, as well as something that will curb your appetite and retain water. On race day I would recommend doubling up your breakfast—oatmeal plus a protein drink. These will give you the nutrition, fluids, and proteins that will carry you through a race.

Finally, toss a couple of single serving bags of nuts in your race bag. Afterward, these will be a great snack providing protein, carbs, fats, and salt.

Week 4.
Daily Workout

Fitness requires physical activity. It requires using the muscles, bones, and tendons that make up 90% of your body, but which get used less than 10% of the day. For most of every day the amazing capabilities of your body are totally ignored and unused. It is impossible to be fit and healthy without using, challenging, and developing that body.

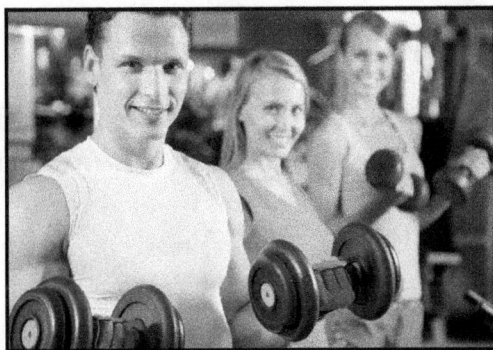

If exercise were education, most people would have only a high school diploma. They stop their active life when childhood play and school sports end. Most people see exercise as something for children, rather than as a permanent part of their adult life from the cradle to the grave. But the fact is that the best way to put distance between your cradle and your grave is to exercise all the way along the road.

In school we get the impression that exercise and sports are just for "the jocks". That is a completely warped picture. Exercise, sports, and physical activity are for everyone who has a body, from the coordinated to the klutz, from the muscular to the skinny, from the outgoing to the introverted. If you have a body, then it needs regular exercise. It is hungry for regular exercise. It grows with exercise and decays without it. In real life, gyms and home exercise programs are for everyone.

Without a healthy and strong body, you compromise your ability to live in every other way as well. A lack of exercise leads to bad moods and poor thinking because the chemistry in your body is messed up. Exercise will help regulate your emotions. It will increase blood and oxygen to the brain, improving your thinking and reasoning. Your body is a biological, chemical, and electrical machine. Thinking and feeling are not separate from moving and sweating. All of this is tied together into a single supportive package. Without exercise you limit everything that happens in your body package.

How Often?

The most common question that people ask about exercise is around how often they should do it.

- How many days per week should I exercise?
- How long should I rest between workouts?

Your body is a fantastic machine that can perform outstanding feats if you use it and train it. For such a wonderful ma-

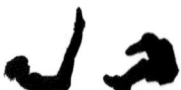

chine, there is a simple answer to how often to exercise. You should only exercise on the same days that you eat. If you do not eat on Saturday's then do not exercise on Saturday's either. But on any day that you consume the calories that fuel your physical body, you should also exercise that body and convert that fuel into muscle, endurance, and flexibility.

Tom says ...

— — —

"Exercise every day that you eat."

— — —

This new thinking is contrary to what many people were taught in decades past. It is also not the "minimum recommended" amount of exercise. Daily exercise is the "optimum recommended" amount.

People try to put exercise into a unique position in their lives. Seldom do they ask:

How many days per week should I eat?
How many days per week should I sleep?
How many days should I learn?
How many days should I bathe?

For all of these they automatically assume that it is every single day. But when it comes to exercise, suddenly they think they need a day or two between workouts to rest and recover.

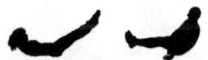

Why does that same rule not apply to sleeping or eating? Applying that rule to Thanksgiving Dinner would mean that we would eat a huge meal on Thursday and then rest from eating for at least two days, or maybe as many as four days. Since it was an "extreme meal" we may not eat again until at least Saturday or Sunday.

Try the same for sleeping. If you have an "extreme sleep" of 12 hours one night, do you decide to rest from sleeping by skipping the next night and running straight through two solid days without sleep?

Certainly not! So why would you do this with exercise?

Exercise is a daily activity. Daily ... as in every day.

Tony Horton, who is famous for promoting the P90X® workout program, says that his exercise plan is to workout every day. He does not plan a day off each week. He plans to exercise on every day that he can and then allows his work and travel schedule to determine when he must skip a day. This insures that he does not double up on days off because he intentionally rested for a day and then found the next day so busy that he was forced to skip a workout because of his schedule. He says that he has often found himself exercising 19 days in a row until he finally hit a travel day that required him to skip one workout. But on a more typical week his schedule will force him to miss one or even two days, so there is no need to intentionally plan a rest day when his normal

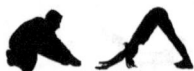

working schedule will do that for him. That is the right approach to scheduling exercise.

If you have a workout every day, then you are also going to need to change up your exercise routines. You cannot do heavy lifting for your chest every single day. That is not conductive to muscle building and it is not a balanced approach to fitness. People who exercise daily have a variety of routines available to choose from, just as most of us have a variety of foods available for different meals. They exercise differently every day, just as they eat different foods every day. This provides interesting variety, prevents overexertion of one muscle group, and creates balance between all of the functions of the body.

INTENSITY

Once you begin exercising every day you will develop a stamina for it that is much higher than people who just exercise three days a week will ever experience. You will also find that you develop a level of energy that is much higher than you are used to. Exercise will cause your body to increase its daily metabolism, which means converting the food that you consume into energy. Many people find that this gives them the energy to work all day long and still tackle the activities that they enjoy afterward.

At the beginning of your new workout program you will experience exhaustion and soreness. But that is a temporary adjustment to a new type of body and a new level of fitness.

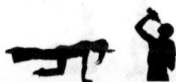

It will pass and you will find that you often have more energy after a workout than you did before. That energy will allow you to spend more time enjoying the rest of your day.

Tom says ...

■■■   ■■■   ■■■

"Before you start a new and vigorous exercise program, you need to consult your physician. Get a physical. Tell your doctor that you are planning to start an exercise program and share this book. Listen to your doctor's concerns and follow his or her guidance. This book will be read by thousands of people. It is a general blueprint for fitness. Only your physician can tell you what your body is really ready to tackle."

■■■   ■■■   ■■■

Since you will be exercising every day, you will need multiple alternating routines. Every day cannot be a 100% exertion day. Some days you may focus on building muscle. Others you will burn fat. Then you will work on cardio or flexibility. I refer to these workout routines as:

- Build—Grow muscle
- Burn—Rip off the fat and water
- Breathe—Stress the cardio vascular system
- Bend—Increase flexibility

Each of these stresses your body and enriches it in a different way.

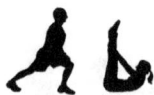

Building muscle can be very taxing. After a tough building workout you may need to rest from that activity for a day or two. But you do not want to do nothing. This is a good time to focus on cardiovascular health with bicycling, running, or swimming; or improve your flexibility with a yoga or martial arts workout.

Personally I get the most energy and the most mental exhilaration from a Burning workout. This is a dynamic moving workout that challenges my muscles with strength moves while keeping me running to build cardio at the same time.

TRAINING COACH

Effective training is based on science. Understanding how the human body operates, grows, and repairs itself is essential for designing effective training programs. The science of fitness makes important advances every year just like the science of computers, biology, and astronomy. If you are going to get the best results, you need to be plugged into the growing body of knowledge about fitness, nutrition, and exercise. What you learned in high school has been improved enormously over the last three decades. Even what you may have learned just five years ago is a little outdated.

You cannot do your best if you are using outdated and ineffective training methods.

You cannot get fit using "your father's workout".

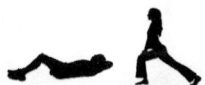

When you look back at the pictures of Olympic athletes from 30, 40, or 50 years ago you notice that their bodies were built very differently from the athletes competing today. They had less muscle mass and more fat. They look more like today's casual high school athletes or the average fit people in any local gym. They did not look like the best athletes in the world.

Those athletes were using the best training programs and nutrition advice that was available to them at the time. They were being advised by scientists, coaches, and other athletes who knew much less about the human body and how to develop its abilities than these same people know today.

If you have not read a fitness book or watched a training DVD in the last 10 years, then you are living in the stone age of physical training and fitness. Older programs prescribed 60 minutes of exercise followed by a full day of rest, usually limiting you to three workouts a week. That is very outdated and much less effective than what you can accomplish today.

Most people believe that they already know how to exercise, eat, hydrate, and take vitamins because they have done each of these at some point in the last 20 years. But they are wrong.

The science of fitness has changed significantly. You should not try to design your own workout program with Build, Burn, Breathe, and Bend all mixed into it. It is much better to find a professional who has done several hundred of these and who has the education to know how to do it effectively.

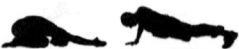

Live human trainers can be very motivating and helpful at developing good habits in the gym. If you are just starting out or are not able to motivate yourself to workout daily, then you should schedule some time with a personal trainer. Let this person evaluate your current level of fitness. Let them design a workout routine that fits your current abilities. Let them show you how to do the exercises and how to use the equipment. Within a few weeks you will be much more comfortable in the gym, more adept at using the equipment, and more aware of what your body can do. Your trainer should be constantly adjusting the routines to fit your abilities and to keep you interested. The investment that you make in a trainer for three or four weeks is generally money well spent.

At the average gym, a trainer will charge between $30 and $75 an hour for a session. At this rate, most people cannot afford to work with them for months or years. Neither should you feel that you have too. Once you are comfortable with your workouts, you should wean yourself off of the trainer and begin to take control of your workouts.

Luckily, there are also world-class trainers who will work with you for months or years at one set price. The recent success of DVD programs like P90X® has triggered a tidal wave of really good training programs of all types. Some of the best trainers in the world have packaged their knowledge into books and DVD's. You can hire them to train you over and over for the same price that you would pay a live person for a single hour. Trainers like Tony Horton, Jackie Warner, Jillian Michaels, Tom Holland, Billy Banks, and Rodney Yee have all produced

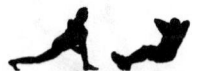

some outstanding materials to personally walk you through their training programs. Give them a chance. The claims that they make in their advertisements are true, they really can transform your body if you follow their programs.

My Modern Exercise Surprise

After decades of designing my own workout routines in the gym, I picked up the Supreme 90 Day® workout program for only $20. I was extremely surprised to find out that exercise routines had evolved a great deal since I had last read about them. I found Tom Holland running through a routine that used relatively light weights, but which was more tasking on my muscles, cardio, and flexibility than I was accomplishing in twice the time with much heavier weights in the gym. By following his new training methods my body quickly became much fitter than I was able to accomplish on my own. My muscles became stronger and more firm. Twenty pounds of fat melted off of my body. My cardio fitness improved significantly and I was much more flexible. My entire body was tied together so that I was better able to play sports and simply sit upright at my office computer. All of this improvement occurred while reducing my workout time from 60 minutes to 40 minutes per day.

I also learned to incorporate variety into my training. The Supreme 90 Day® program, and other like it, incorporates weight training, calisthenics, cardio, yoga, and stretching. These are much richer and healthier workouts than I had been practicing on my own. I was especially surprised to find

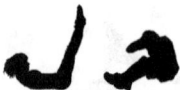

the modern emphasis on strong core training and its ability to create six-pack abs for normal people.

This experience made me a believer in modern advances in fitness, training, and nutrition. From this foundation I began to explore workouts and diets from the other trainers listed in this book and found that the entire approach to fitness had changed since I last studied it to create my old workouts. With these methods I was able to remain more fit using shorter, more intense workouts.

Hiring help from a personal trainer, from a DVD, or from a book will pay huge dividends.

EXERCISE PROGRAMS

Build ■ Burn ■ Breathe ■ Bend

Tom Says ...

— — —

"When you pick a workout for the day, it should accomplish one of four fitness objectives: Build Muscle, Burn Fat, Breathe Deep (Cardio), or Bend Over (Flexibility). During any given week you should combine workouts that address at least two or three of these."

— — —

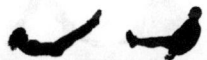

This book is a little different in that it does not contain 100 pages of pictures of people exercising. Most authors feel obligated to demonstrate all of the exercises that they recommend and to write an explanation of the form, movement, weight, and muscles targeted.

Those picture sections are useful for identifying new exercises to put into your own gym routine. But they are not the best way to design and run your daily workouts. The best approach is to hire a personal trainer or to buy a personal trainer on DVD. Either one of these will give you a well designed workout program and lead you through it every day. This approach is much better than trying to piece together your own from pictures in a book.

Therefore, my approach to a new blueprint for fitness is to point you to some of the best trainers in the world and to recommend that you spend a small amount of money to purchase one of their DVD sets and use it daily. This is a great way to get started on a new path. These programs will provide the intensity, variety, and motivation that you need to stick with a daily workout program and to learn all of the new ideas that are effective for improving your fitness.

These videos should include routines that Build Muscle—Burn Fat—Breathe Cardio—and Bend Flexibility. Most of those that we recommend accomplish all of this for less than $20.

- Supreme 90 Day® Workout—My favorite for intensity, variety, and high energy.

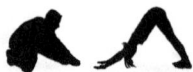

- P90X®—The best selling program in the country.
- Jackie Warner's Power Circuit Training—Five different workouts on one DVD.
- Jackie Warner's Xtreme Timesaver Training®—A great full body workout in 30 minutes.
- Jillian Michaels' 30 Day Solution®—Intense workouts with one of the most popular trainers in the world.
- Rodney Yee's Power Yoga—For flexibility, balance, muscle tone, and relaxation.
- Beachbody 10 Minute Trainer®—For those times when you just have a few minutes to squeeze in a workout.
- 10 Minute Solution®: Pilates—Great stretching routines to increase flexibility and reduce stress.
- Weider's X-Factor: ST®—Full body workouts that require no weights or equipment.
- Barry's Boot Camp®—High energy workout with elastic bands and a stability ball.

These are just a few of the excellent programs available. Each is affordable and approachable. Feel free to experiment. If you love the first one you try, then stick with it for a few months or a year. If it does not groove for you, then try one of the others.

Most people have a dozen pairs of shoes in the closet. There are the black and brown dress shoes, the daily tennis shoes and the running shoes, the old yard shoes and the slippers. Fitness programs are a lot like your shoes. One program may not meet every need that you have. You may need some that are long, some short, some cardio, some with weights, and

some for stretching. The multi-DVD sets try to do all of these in one package and generally do a great job of it.

The Supreme 90 Day® DVD set is my standard daily workout. But when I need variety I will use a Jackie Warner video to change the pace. Once a week I go through a 60 minute yoga routine to stretch my muscles, improve my posture, and develop my balance.

There is no reason to limit yourself to a single style of workout. Just use the ones that fit your day and your style. But do something every day.

INTENSITY LEVEL

Each of the videos I have listed has a different intensity level. You should choose one that is a step above where your fitness level is right now. The Smithfield Scale of Workout Intensity shows roughly where each product falls in intensity and hard work. When a set contains multiple workouts, some will be much higher intensity than others. For example, Jackie Warner is known for her intense abdominal workouts. So even though her cardio workout may rate about a 7, her abdominal workouts are closer to 9. X-Factor:ST® is very strong in cardio, perhaps an 8, while its muscle building is closer to a 5 or 6.

After using Supreme 90 Day® for nine months I had mastered every workout in the set—except one. The Tabata Inferno workout was designed with 20 seconds or work and

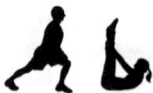

10 seconds of rest for 8 cycles. The entire workout includes several of these circuits to create a 30 minute workout that is extremely cardio challenging. Even after a year I found that this routine could tax me to my limits. The only way I could stay on top of it was to do it at least once a week. So, even though I rated the product an 8 overall, I would give the Tabata Inferno workout a 9 or 10.

Use the Smithfield scale as guidance in getting started, but expect some surprises in each DVD set. They are all filled with challenges.

The Smithfield Scale of Workout Intensity

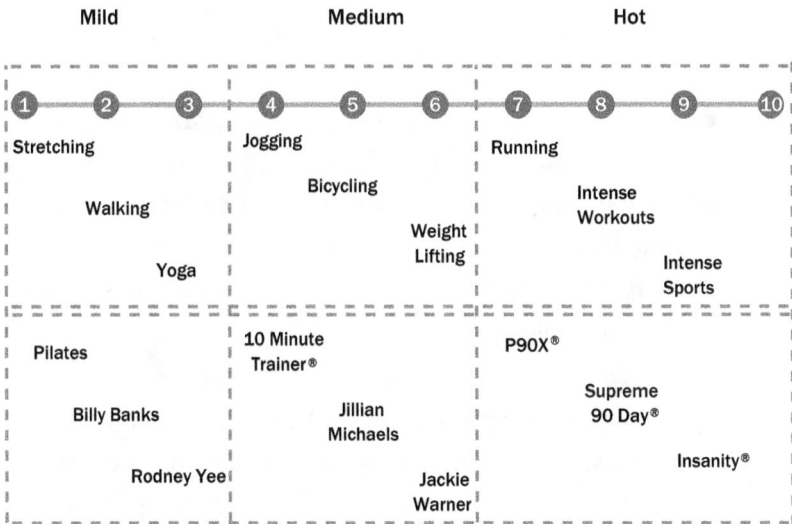

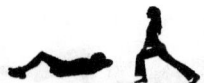

Mild	Medium	Hot

① ② ③	④ ⑤ ⑥	⑦ ⑧ ⑨ ⑩
Stretching	Jogging	Running
	Bicycling	
Walking		Intense Workouts
	Weight Lifting	
Yoga		Intense Sports
Pilates	10 Minute Trainer®	P90X®
		Supreme 90 Day®
Billy Banks	Jillian Michaels	
		Insanity®
Rodney Yee	Jackie Warner	

ACCESSORIES

Do you need expensive equipment and expensive clothes to do a good workout? Definitely not!

Your workout equipment should cost about what you would spend for a professional outfit for work. Add up the price of a pair of shoes, socks, pants, shirt, tie, and underwear. The amount that you spent on this one set of clothes is a generous budget for workout equipment.

I would recommend the following pieces of equipment to match the exercise DVD's listed:

- Light Dumbbells—5 to 10 pounds for women, 10 to 20 pounds for men.
- Inflatable Stability Ball—a great platform for hundreds of exercises.
- Elastic Band—a simple flat noodle band that can be folded to increase resistance.
- Yoga Mat—put this down if your floors are too dirty to be exercising on.

That is enough to get you started and to keep you going for many months. Once you have your momentum you may want to add to this collection. But in the beginning do not throw too much money around.

For clothing you need some loose fitting shirts and shorts that will allow you to breathe, but also collect the sweat. A

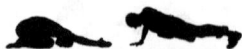

basic t-shirt and exercise shorts are fine. Some people prefer to get non-cotton materials to reduce the amount of sweat that collects and to allow more air circulation.

For shoes, any pair of sport shoe will work for the DVD's listed. You are not going to be running a marathon or lifting iron that is twice your body weight. You do not need special shoes, just something comfortable and well fitting to your foot.

Use the "price of a set of professional clothing" rule for the amount you might spend on workout clothes as well.

PICKING THE BEST WORKOUT VIDEOS

After using all of the DVDs described in this chapter, as well as many that are not listed, I definitely have my favorites. These are the ones that I turn to every week, which are effective and interesting enough to follow for months at a time.

My Favorite Workout Videos

Total Workout Plan	10 Minute Workout
Supreme 90 Day® Jackie Warner Power Circuit Training®	10 Minute Trainer® Jackie Warner Power Circuit Training®
Abs Only	Yoga
X-Factor: ST® Supreme 90 Day®	Rodney Yee X-Factor: ST®

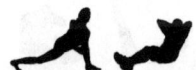

You will find pros and cons to each of these workouts.

Supreme 90 Day®

- ♨ **Pro:** Great intensity. Great muscle building. Moderate equipment requirement. Very thorough.
- ☞ **Con:** No Yoga or flexibility workout.

Jackie Warner Power Circuit Training®

- ♨ **Pro:** Five tough workouts on one DVD. Very tough core routines.
- ☞ **Con:** Not enough variety for a year-long workout plan.

10 Minute Trainer®

- ♨ **Pro:** Short, fun, and intense. Great for Morning Metabolism Boost. Lots of variety in eight workouts.
- ☞ **Con:** Not long enough to be your main workout for the day.

X-Factor:ST®

- ♨ **Pro:** Great intensity. Strong emphasis on cardio and core.
- ☞ **Con:** Weak on muscle building, especially upper body.

Rodney Yee Power Yoga

- ♨ **Pro:** Great yoga flexibility, muscle building, and tension release.
- ☞ **Con:** Moderate intensity for fat burning.

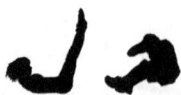

Barry's Boot Camp®

- 👍 **Pro:** High energy, fat burning routines. Minimal equipment required.
- 👎 **Con:** No yoga or stretching. Limited muscle building.

These are just some tips to help you pick a program that meets your needs in the beginning. Over time you will develop your own preferences, but by then you will not need my help because you will be successfully working on your own.

KNOWING AND DOING

In the 21st century, most people know a lot about fitness and nutrition. You see it on television, in magazines, in newspaper columns, and hear it from all of our friends. So you already know more about exercise than you are putting into practice. The goal of this chapter is not to teach you more about exercise, but to point you in a direction that will get you to **do** more.

DVD's or live human trainers are two of the best ways to get you to move from thinking about exercise, to doing it every day.

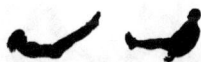

WEEKLY SHOPPING LIST

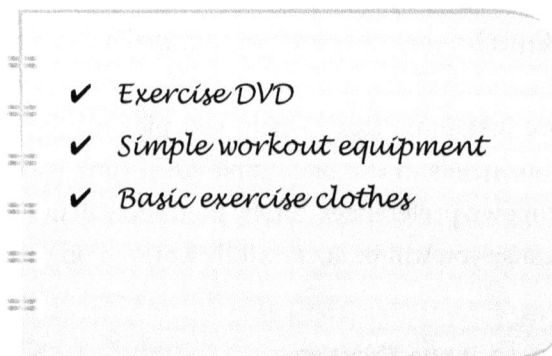

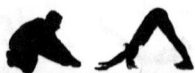

✔ Exercise DVD

✔ Simple workout equipment

✔ Basic exercise clothes

Mud 4.
Grimy Workout

Mud runs are a full-body work out. You need the strength to pull yourself over walls, flexibility to contort through obstacles, cardio to run the entire race, and stamina to recover quickly between challenges.

The high intensity interval training that is recommended in this Blueprint combines all of these features in your weekly training. Variety and intensity are the best combinations to prepare for a mud run. Each day's workout should challenge your body in a new way. Switch between strength building, cardio vascular, flexibility, and metabolism burning workouts. Each day should be as intense as you can make it.

I do best when I put all types of workouts into the week immediately before a mud run. Then the day before the event I dial it back to a modest workout. This might include a ten minute morning metabolism boost and a short run. Since running is a core part of a mud run, keeping my cardio active the day before a run makes my lungs more efficient on the day of the run. My goal on that final day is to keep my body primed, but allow it to store up the energy it needs for the race.

Here is one good workout program for the week before a mud run.

Day	Focus	Sample Workouts
Monday	Strength	• Jackie Warner 30 Day Fast Start—Upper Body • Supreme 90 Day—Check & Back
Tuesday	Strength	• Jackie Warner 30 Day Fast Start—Lower Body • Supreme 90 Day—Legs • Add: Supreme 90 Day—Rock Hard Abs
Wednesday	Cardio	• Supreme 90 Day—Tabata Inferno • Jillian Michaels Extreme Shed and Shred Level 2
Thursday	Burn	• Bob Harper's Inside-Out—"Bob's Workout"
Friday	Prime	• Morning Metabolism plus a Short Run
Saturday	Mud Run	• Get Dirty!
Sunday	Stretching	• Bob Harper's Inside-Out—Yoga • P90X2—Yoga

RUNNING

Following any daily workout, you may want to add a one to three mile run to get your heart, lungs, and legs ready for the big event. If you want to get your performance times down, there is no substitute for daily runs.

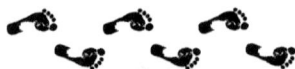

CORE

Most courses include walls, monkey bars, and rope climbs. These appear to be arm and back challenges. But they also call for a strong core to pull your lower body up and other as well. A weak core is a key reason that many people struggle with these obstacles. If you include a short 10-20 minute core exercise in your workouts every other day, you will have chiseled abs and a secret ingredient for beating some of the toughest obstacles. Jackie Warner's workouts have some of the best core routines that I have tried.

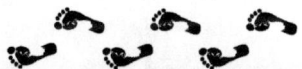

WEEK 5.
POWER PROTEIN DRINKS

The most difficult nutrient to get into your body every day is protein. Vitamins and minerals can be dropped in as a pill every morning. Water runs from every tap in the country. Carbohydrates come with every piece of fruit and have been packed into every processed food item on the store shelves. Then there is the fat ... who needs more of that? But protein typically requires a specific decision to base a meal on meat, chicken, fish, soy, nuts, or beans. Doing this for at least two meals a day every day can be difficult. Also, most

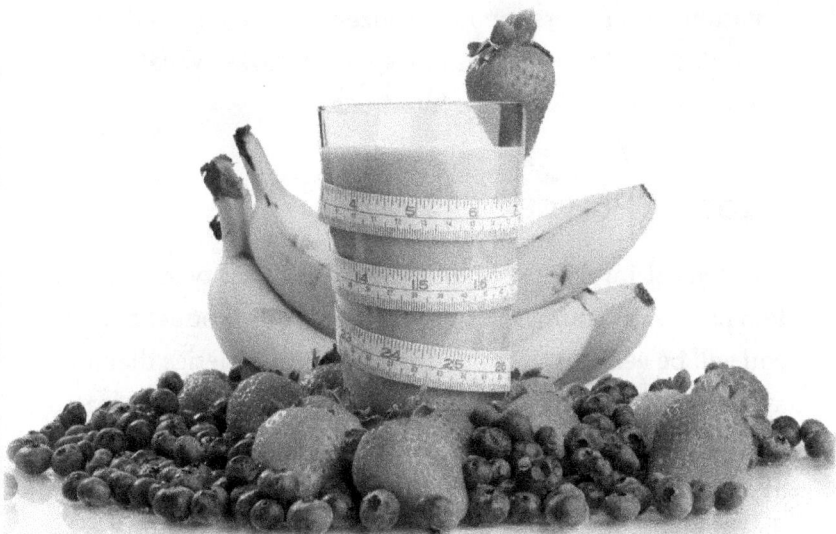

meat recipes include too much fat and salt along with the protein that they provide.

The best solution for this problem is to incorporate home-made protein drinks into your diet. The ones that we recommend will also deliver a healthy dose of fiber and complex carbohydrates. They are so filling and nutritious that they can serve as an entire meal.

Protein drinks are a lot like Mexican food. They use the same ingredients prepared in many different combinations. Beans, meat, tortillas, cheese, lettuce, tomatoes, and sauce can make tacos, burritos, enchiladas, tostadas, quesadillas, and a dozen other dishes.

The same is true of protein drinks. Protein powder, milk, juice, fruit, yogurt, nut butter, and oatmeal in different combinations and flavors can make dozens of different and delicious drinks. Add in cinnamon, spinach leaves, wheat germ, and flax seeds and you have hundreds.

PROTEIN POWDER

The central ingredient to all of these is some type of protein powder. If you have not shopped for this product before you will be very surprised at the number of varieties that are available. Every grocery and discount store carries at least half a dozen different products. A health food store may have as many as a hundred products. They offer protein that is derived from milk, egg, whey, soy, hemp, and other bizarre

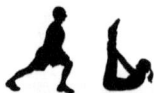

ingredients. Then there are dozens of different flavors and "nutritional boosters".

Most of the specialized products are for people with very unique training needs. They are not for the average consumer. Ninety percent of the people working on their health and fitness can choose a product based on four simple criteria.

1. **Sugar-free.** Choose a powder without significant added sugar, preferably no added sugar at all. You can figure this out simply by reading the label. Do the ingredients list any form of sugar? You can also look at the Carbohydrates per serving. If there are more grams of carbs in a serving than there are grams of protein, then don't touch it.

2. **Flavor.** Protein powders are available in almost as many flavors as ice cream. The most popular are plain (no flavor added at all), vanilla, and chocolate. For my own needs I use all three of these. More on that later.

3. **Isolate or Concentrate.** Concentrated protein is similar to dehydrated milk. It is a product like milk, egg, or soy from which the water content has been removed and the remaining material has been turned into a powder. Isolated protein takes this a step further by removing almost all material which is not a protein. As a result, the isolate product usually has more protein and fewer carbs per serving. It is also generally more expensive. I would recommend choosing an isolate product if the slightly higher price is not an issue for you.

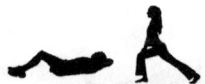

4. **Lactose.** Many people have at least a mild form of lactose intolerance. The best way to get protein powder without lactose is to choose one made from soy. The soy also has other valuable health benefits. If your own lactose intolerance is mild, then you can also choose a whey isolate product. These are very close to being entirely lactose free. Read the label to be sure.

If you answer these four simple questions you will narrow your search down to a few basic products. From those you can experiment until you find the one with a taste, texture, and "mixability" that you prefer.

Entire books have been written on supplementation and the detailed contents and properties of protein powder. I think it is much better to answer the four basic questions and begin to experiment for yourself. You should also engage the store clerks in conversation. They have tried many of the products and can be a big help if you already know what you expect in the area of sugar, flavor, composition, and lactose.

Tom says ...

— — —

"Protein powder varies greatly in price. But the basic contents of all of the products are similar. If you can find a mixture that you like at a bargain price, then go for it. I like the plain soy and whey isolate products without any boosters or fancy additives."

— — —

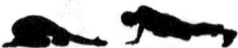

Meal and Snack

Nutrition rich protein drinks are not a liquid that will replace water, tea, or soda in a meal. They are meals and snacks on their own. These drinks infuse your body with protein, carbohydrates, healthy fats, and fiber. They are so rich with nutrition that they are more powerful than most of the foods you can order in a restaurant. For one dollar or less, the nutrition in these is equal to the nutrition of a meal that would cost ten to fifteen dollars.

Each day you can choose to drink one, two, or three of these powerful mixtures. One may be breakfast, the next an afternoon snack, and the last a post-workout recovery drink.

These drinks will taste so good that you are tempted to think of them as milk shakes or deserts. There is no harm in that. It is quite a complement to a food that you are able to make yourself. But be careful that you do not turn that thinking around and start substituting a desert for your protein drink.

Mixers and Blenders

I have one protein smoothie for breakfast every morning and a second following my afternoon workout. That means I need a mixer at home and another in my office. I have a nice blender at home, but I hate to clean the equipment at work, so like thousands of other people, I use a shaker cup at work. When you are looking for a device to mix up your smoothies, you can find something very effective at a low price.

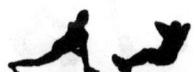

There are a few basic categories of mixers that will meet most of your needs.

1. **Traditional Blender.** These can handle about two quarts of liquids and ingredients. They have the power to chop and liquefy all fruits, vegetables, and powders. If you are blending for two people these are ideal.

2. **Magic Bullet®.** This is the perfect single serving mixer. You blend and drink from the same cup. It is small and compact. It is easy to clean. It comes with multiple cups and blender heads so you always have a clean one when some are in the dishwasher. It has almost all of the power of a traditional blender. This is the workhorse tool for my daily morning smoothie.

3. **Traditional Mini Blender.** This small version of a traditional blender is inexpensive and very portable. It works best with liquids and powders, but is a little under-powered for chopping up fruits and vegetables. It can be very handy for a simple liquid and powder smoothie.

4. **Protein Shaker Cup.** Most health food stores and grocery stores sell "shaker cups" right next to their selection of protein powders. These require no electricity. They are powered by the human arm. Some include a blending device inside, like a propeller in the cap or a little spring ball that bounces around inside when you are shaking. Obviously these cannot chop fruit, but they are 100% portable and can be used on the spot to mix powders and liquids.

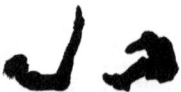

Gym rats carry these in their bags and mix up a drink in the locker room immediately after a workout.

5. **Spaghetti Sauce Jar.** If you want to go old school you can use a spaghetti sauce jar as a shaker cup. These have the advantage of being nearly free and being disposable if they get a little to smelly. Since these jars are meant to store acidic tomato-based spaghetti sauce, they are made from sturdy glass with a lid that has an excellent seal that prevents rust and corrosion. They can be washed repeatedly in the dishwasher. Some of these jars are real works of art and it is a shame to discard them once the sauce is gone. Repurposing them as your protein drink mixer is a nice eco-conscious solution. Also, since they are nearly free, you can have three or four of them in the food drawer of your desk at work. If you carry one home, there are more waiting to be used the next day.

I am a big fan of the Magic Bullet® and the Spaghetti Sauce jar. My coworkers have gotten used to seeing me walking down the hall shaking a glass mason jar filled with chocolate liquid. They don't ask questions anymore, but kindly act like it is totally normal.

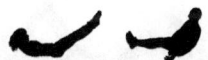

STARTER KIT

As I said earlier, protein drinks are like Mexican food, a lot of recipes come from the same basic ingredients. Small changes in the mixture can lead to interesting and delicious flavors. I am including a couple of my favorite combinations in this chapter. But, it is important that you experiment for yourself. Find the flavors that most appeal to you. As long as you are using healthy ingredients, do not be afraid to throw your imagination into the blender.

Jackie Warner is a world famous trainer whose body is fit, trim, and powerful. But, in spite of her devotion to health and nutrition, she admits that she really hates eating spinach. It is a valuable food that just never appealed to her taste buds. Rather than avoiding spinach leaves, she puts them into her daily protein drinks for a "green protein smoothie". The spinach taste is masked by all of the other ingredients. Their texture is chopped and covered with liquid. But their nutrition is still 100% in the drink. You can do the same with any of the important and powerful foods that you just cannot force yourself to eat plain, raw, or alone.

GREAT INGREDIENTS IN YOUR KITCHEN

To be consistent with these protein drinks, you need to stock up on the ingredients, both at home and at work. Add the following to your next grocery shopping trip.

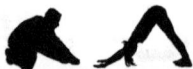

- *Milk.* Choose something low fat that meets your dietary needs. If you have a lactose problem, then use lactose free dairy, soy, or almond milk.

- *Fruit Juice.* Be sure to use juice with no added sugar. This is going to give you a lot of color, sweetness, and volume. Dole® has a number of great choices that you can use to change up these recipes.

- *Plain Greek Yogurt.* If you can stand the lactose, this yogurt will add a thickness that is very nice. Do not use the flavored ones because they have a lot of sugar.

- *Ground Flax Seed.* This will give your smoothie a nutty flavor. The fiber will also improve your digestion and clean your intestines.

- *Natural Nut Butter.* Grocery stores usually carry peanut and almond butters without added sugar. Health food stores have a dozen different nut butters. My favorite is sunflower seed butter. It has a richer flavor than the peanut, with a unique punch that is refreshing.

- *Cinnamon.* Recent studies have shown several health benefits of cinnamon. This led to it showing up on the supplement aisles in capsule form. But this ingredient is so cheap that you should just get a big shaker of it and add liberally to your drinks and morning oatmeal.

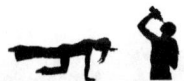

- *Oatmeal.* I like to make my smoothies a little thicker and give them more complex carbohydrates by adding a spoonful or two of plain oatmeal. This helps boost the drink to the level of a meal that easily replaces what most people eat in the morning.

- *Spinach Leaves.* Jackie Warner's trick may sound strange, but if you give it a try you will find that a vegetable-based smoothie can be as delicious as one based on fruit.

- *Bottled Iced Tea.* Several companies make some wonderful flavors of healthy and sugar-free teas. These can be the basis for a very refreshing and lighter protein smoothie. Just crack the top and pour in about half a bottle.

- *Mio® Flavor Drops.* This product is new to most stores. It is designed to give flavor to water bottles. One of them also contains caffeine if this is part of your diet.

- *Liquid Protein.* These are the protein shots that you find in vitamin shops and some convenience stores. When creating a smoothie based on iced tea, a protein powder can ruin the light texture so you can substitute one of these shots. Choose one without extra "Energy", which means a high caffeine content.

These are just some of the ingredients that you might want to keep on hand near your blender. Experiment for yourself and find others that you enjoy.

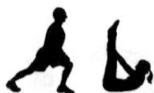

GREAT SMOOTHIE RECIPES

Fruit Boost	Veggie Boost
Soy or Almond Milk—½ cup	Soy or Almond Milk—½ cup
Fruit Juice—½ cup	Vegetable Juice—½ cup
Greek Yogurt—1 tablespoon	Spinach Leaves—5 or 6 leaves
Fruit—Half	Plain Protein Power—1 scoop
Plain Protein Power—1 scoop	Ground Flax Seed—1 spoonful
Ground Flax Seed—1 spoonful	Natural Nut Butter—1 spoonful
Natural Nut Butter—1 spoonful	
Cinnamon—big shake	
Oatmeal—1 spoonful	
Power Tea	**Protein Quencher**
Snapple® Diet Tea—½ bottle	Filtered Water
Liquid Protein	Flavored Protein Powder
Ground Flax Seed	Mio® Flavor Drops
	Ground Flax Seed

That last Protein Quencher is easy to make in a shaker cup or spaghetti sauce jar. It is ideal at work or as a post-workout smoothie.

Finally, there are a number of bottled protein drinks that you can get in stores. Some of these have excellent ingredients and great flavors. But I find that most of them are too expensive to recommend as a regular daily drink. You can make something with more nutrition for a quarter of the price of these bottled drinks. Also, the inexpensive ones are generally little more than milk and sugar. I would recommend using

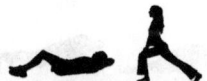

these only when you are unable to make your own, but do not lean on them as your daily mainstay.

Protein smoothies are like discovering a new ethnic restaurant. There are a lot of great flavors to explore and enjoy.

WEEKLY SHOPPING LIST

✔ Protein Powder
✔ Milk (Low-fat Dairy, Almond, Soy, or Lactose-free)
✔ Fresh Fruit
✔ 100% Fruit Juice
✔ Plain Greek Yogurt
✔ Ground Flax Seed
✔ Natural Nut Butter
✔ Cinnamon Shaker
✔ Diet Bottled Teas

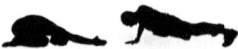

MUD 5.
MONKEY PROTEIN DRINKS

In the Blueprint Fitness chapter you learned that the American diet is far too short on good, lean, healthy protein. Because simple carbs and fats are so tasty and cheap to purchase, most of the prepared food items are heavy on those ingredients. These can be good for quick energy, but they cannot be the basis for building a strong, performance body. Your muscles are made from protein. To create the muscle strength that you need for mud running, you have to fuel your body with protein.

I recommend a protein drink every morning and possibly a second in the afternoon following a workout. For an active athlete and people who want to improve their mud run performance, the second protein drink is not optional. You definitely need the fuel and building blocks every day.

WEEK 6.
RECHARGE & RENEW

We live our daily lives like we use our cell phones—always on. From the moment that we arise in the morning until we drop onto the bed at night, we spend almost every moment accomplishing something. We are addicted to activity. We view each minute as an opportunity to get one or two more things done. Life has become a frantic exercise in checking items off of a permanent To Do list.

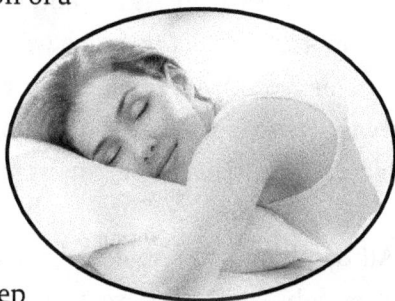

Constant activity like this leaves little room for rest, recovery, reflection, and recharging. Most of us believe that minimizing sleep and down-time is a sign of power and success. It is a measure of how successful we are now and will become in the future. But, this view is short sighted. It assumes that we each have an infinite pool of energy to draw from. Somehow we expect to constantly drain energy out and never refill our internal reservoirs.

Jack Groppel has challenged this by comparing life to running. He asks, "Is life a sprint or a marathon?" Many people describe it as a marathon in which you need to keep running for 30 or 40 years. So you build endurance for long periods of running. Groppel sees it differently. He believes life is a series of sprints. Each day is made up of several sprinting sessions. Between each of these you need to rest and recover. His recipe, and that of the Human Performance Institute, is to break the day into several 90 to 120 minute segments. During each of these you are charged up for a working sprint with maximum energy. At the end of this period you must recharge your energy for 5 to 20 minutes in preparation for the next sprint.

If you use this method, you will find that you have plenty of energy for work at the end of the day, just as you did in the morning. Most people have high energy and focus in the morning, followed by an exhausting afternoon fueled by caffeine. There is a healthier and more sustainable pattern if you incorporate rest and nutritious snacks throughout the day.

All day long you should be recharging with healthy foods, stretch breaks, mild exercises, breathing, and walking. You do not let your body and mind run so long that they are exhausted beyond your ability to recover quickly.

In modern business society, the use of rest breaks is rarely supported. Dedication is demonstrated by unrelenting effort for eight, or ten, or twelve hours a day. This model appears to be very productive for the company, but it is disastrous for the human mind and body. It drives people to drink too much caffeine, eat a poor diet filled with sugary snack foods,

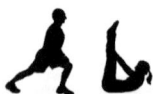

overuse alcohol for relaxation, over medicate, and sleep too little.

If you make the decision to recharge yourself throughout the day, you may have to keep this practice a secret. It might require masking these breaks as an extra trip to the restroom, a walk across the building to see a coworker, a return to your car for something that you forgot to bring in, or a closed door session for a short imaginary telecon. If your organization is not supportive of midday recovery, you need to be creative to practice it.

REST SNACK

Just as your schedule includes standard meals and smaller snacks to keep your energy high throughout the day, you should have multiple rest breaks during the day. For most of us, we are not talking about a 20 minute nap at our desks. That would be a guaranteed ticket to unemployment.

Instead, your mind and body just need a couple of minutes to shift gears from the main focus of your work toward something that is restorative, relaxing, rewarding, and stimulating. Every 90 to 120 minutes you need to push back from your work and take a "rest snack". The goal of this short break is to release tension, refuel your body, break mental blocks, stimulate circulation, and build up your energy supply so you can be more fully alert and engaged for your next 90 minute sprint.

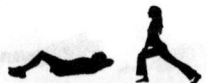

There are literally hundreds of variations on this break. The best usually include a change of scenery, posture, and breathing. For example, get up from your desk and walk up and down two flights of stairs to get a bottle of water and a piece of fruit for a snack. This will change your posture from sitting to standing. It will increase your breathing and circulation from the exertion of walking the stairs. It will boost your energy with the fruit snack. It will give your mind a few minutes to fly free, to see the outside world, and to talk with real people.

Tom says ...

— — —

"The best breaks incorporate:
- Movement and Exertion
- New Location
- Healthy Snack
- Hydration
- Contact with People or Nature"

— — —

If you are in a situation which prohibits leaving your workstation, then you can close your eyes and visualize a break. Since your imagination is doing the work you are not limited to the immediate area around you. Your mental break may include a hike up your favorite mountain or through the woods. It might be a quick swim in the ocean or parachuting

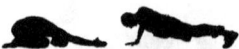

from an airplane. With your eyes closed and your mind still, these imagined breaks can be very effective.

We all have a unique working environment, but there is usually some way for you to include two of these restorative breaks in your daily routine.

My job at the hospital presents constant demands to either work on my computer or attend meetings. Switching between these two activities is a good time to take a restorative break by walking a longer route to the meeting location. This might take me through the cafeteria to pick up a bowl of oatmeal, a piece of fruit, or a bottle of water. When spending long periods at the computer I might visit the kitchen for water and a snack, or step outside to breathe fresh air and circulate my blood. Work tasks are usually unrelenting and constant, so taking a break has to be a conscious decision. Work is not designed to encourage breaks. So you have to design your own habits for recharging, resting, and restoring your energy during the day.

I am especially sympathetic to teachers and nurses. These professions are typically tightly scheduled and focused on meeting the needs of a large number of other people. Often, they literally have no time to use the restroom. My wife jokes about having a teacher's bladder. Their breaks between classes are filled with students who need to ask questions, so they cannot get away for a basic human function until the lunch period and not again until the school day is over.

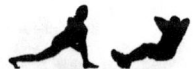

A nurse's schedule can be even tighter. They are constantly responsible for patients, records, and communications with their coworkers. Often it is impossible for them to get away during an entire 8 to 12 hour shift. They have no time to grab a bottle of water and a snack. So they live in a constant state of slight dehydration and low blood sugar. Finding the time to take a break for your biological and mental health is something that your hospital needs to work out with you and all of the nurses. My best advice is to carry a bottle of water, a protein or nutrition bar, and a picture of peace with you at all times. Your breaks are going to happen in seconds rather than minutes.

CYCLIC PATTERN

Here is a simple break plan for a typical day:

7:50 am—Arrive at work. Park near the trees and walk in to the office from there, especially if this is further than your normal parking spot.

10:00 am—Get up from the computer and walk around the halls of the office to visit the water fountain, kitchen, or a friendly coworker. Eat a small snack to restore your energy.

12:00 pm—Prepare for lunch. If you brought your food, take it to a location away from your desk and eat in a natural setting. Incorporate other people into this break if possible.

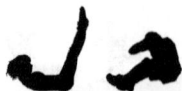

2:00 pm—Go outside with a piece of fruit and bottle of water. Consume your small snack outside before returning to your work. Walk up and down several flights of stairs on your way to and from the outside.

4:00 pm—Push back from your work, close your eyes, and breathe deeply. Spend just 60 seconds clearing your mind, releasing tension, and imagining a tranquil setting. Include some standing muscle stretches at your desk.

5:30 pm—Break for the day. Go for your daily exercise routine.

When you sum up all of these breaks, they are just about 15 or 20 minutes, excluding the lunch break. But the restorative power that these provide will more than compensate for the short work stoppage that occurs. You will find yourself more relaxed at the end of the day, performing more efficiently throughout the day, and more effective in your activities because you have more energy and less stress.

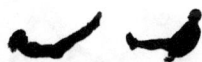

Nature Break

If you have the opportunity, take a nature break every day. I do not mean a trip to the restroom. I mean get outside where you can see, hear, smell, and touch the natural world. Look for an area with trees and grass. These often attract insects and small animals that will divert your attention from work for a brief moment.

Humans have always been a part of the natural world. But we have constructed boxes that separate us from it most of the time. Though these boxes are filled with fascinating, exciting, and satisfying experiences, they do not meet our core need to connect with nature. This is something that we all have to make a conscious effort to maintain.

Workaholic Stubbornness

Workaholics find these ideas very difficult to swallow. They are determined that constant and unrelenting work is the best way to spend every day. Japanese white collar workers are famous for this attitude. They are also famous for mid-career breakdowns which lead to heart attacks on the job and suicide. Chinese factory workers have become famous for working so hard that they leap from high windows to their deaths to escape the energy-draining, soul-grinding life at work. In response, one company installed suicide nets around the building to catch their bodies before they went splat on the pavement. You know you are working too hard in a toxic environment when your health care plan includes suicide nets.

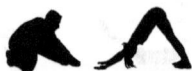

Your mind and body were made to cycle back and forth between focused effort and deliberate relaxation. You cannot alter this cycle through force of will without eventually suffering the consequences of violating the nature of your own mind and body.

Find ways to work with your body, to maintain and grow it so that your life becomes more rewarding and productive. Stop fighting against your nature because society has created an artificial mold that does not work well for the human animal. Look for ways to be more human in your work and personal life, not less human.

Sleep

When we are young, our goal seems to be to stay up as late as possible, but then sleep as long as we can through the morning. Once we get a job, it severely limits our ability to sleep late every morning. But we still try to fit as much into the evening as possible and postpone sleep just a little longer.

What are we trying to accomplish that is so important? Often it is just watching one more television program.

Imagine consciously deciding to go to bed earlier just because you believe that your mind and body need the time to rest, unwind, and recharge. That idea is completely foreign to people who are running their lives by a To Do list or the television schedule. Sleep seems like a waste of valuable time. But this is actually backward. The regeneration that you ex-

perience from sleep will increase your physical and mental wellbeing all day long. It will open up your mind to more creative and productive thoughts than constantly pushing your mind to work late into the night.

Your mind is the seat of your intelligence. But most people treat the mind the way they would a child. If it is not constantly watched, controlled, and guided they fear that it will become lazy and unproductive. But, your mind is completely aware of the problems that you are consciously trying to solve. When you stop pushing it consciously, it continues to work on those same problems at the subconscious level. That is where many of those "Aha!" moments come from in your life. The unexpected solution to a problem emerges from a rested and distracted mind that has been allowed to move problem solving to a new place in the brain, to work at a different pace, and to use a different style than we apply when consciously controlling our thoughts.

Tom says ...

— — —

"Your mind and your body need six to eight hours of sleep each night to heal, to relax, and to recharge for the next day. You cannot rob your body of that sleep and make up for it with coffee the next day, or longer rest on the weekend. Your body has a cycle that includes the need for sleep every day."

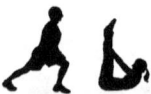

— — —

If you skip a night of sleep or severely shortchange yourself. It is just like skipping several meals. When you finally do sleep you are going to "oversleep" in the same way that you often overeat after missing a meal. When you finally do sit down to a meal in a famished state you often choose foods that are very unhealthy. You eat too much and eat too quickly. Afterward you do not feel recharged, instead you still feel terrible, but now with a full stomach.

When you hit the bed, exhausted from lack of rest, it is actually more difficult to unwind into a relaxed state and drift off to sleep. That is why people who work extremely hard find that they need drugs to help them sleep in spite of the fact that they are exhausted. Exhaustion is not the ideal state to induce sleep. Relaxation is the ideal entry into sleep.

THE SCIENCE OF SLEEP

Sleep is a heightened anabolic state in which growth and rejuvenation of the immune, nervous, skeletal and muscular systems occur. Most animals have a sleep pattern which is a regular part of their lifecycle. In general, the optimal amount of sleep is not a meaningful concept. Rather it is the time at which sleep occurs that is most important. Your body has circadian rhythms which are based on sleep occurring at specific points in that cycle. The sleep that you get at the "wrong time" can be ineffective and inadequate, even when the total number of hours is sufficient. Most importantly, you should be asleep at least six hours before your lowest body temperature of the day. This usually occurs at 4:30am for a person on a

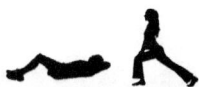

regular circadian clock schedule. That means that you should go to bed by 10:30pm each evening in order to maximize the effectiveness of the sleep hours that you get every day.

The circadian rhythm diagram illustrates the optimum performance times for a wide variety of activities throughout a normal day.

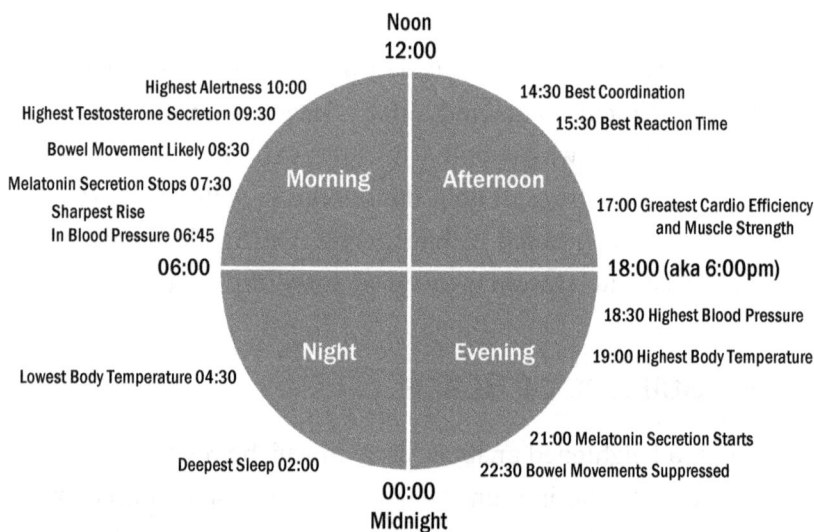

Noon
12:00

Highest Alertness 10:00
Highest Testosterone Secretion 09:30
Bowel Movement Likely 08:30
Melatonin Secretion Stops 07:30
Sharpest Rise
In Blood Pressure 06:45
06:00

14:30 Best Coordination
15:30 Best Reaction Time

17:00 Greatest Cardio Efficiency
and Muscle Strength
18:00 (aka 6:00pm)
18:30 Highest Blood Pressure
19:00 Highest Body Temperature

Morning   Afternoon

Night   Evening

Lowest Body Temperature 04:30

Deepest Sleep 02:00

21:00 Melatonin Secretion Starts
22:30 Bowel Movements Suppressed

00:00
Midnight

Your need for sleep varies throughout your life. The best way for you to measure whether you are getting enough sleep is to notice whether you are drowsy or dysfunctional during the day. If you are receiving six to eight hours of sleep each night, you should be fully functional throughout the day. However, modern office workers have such a sedentary working style that they often find themselves sleepy or daydreaming in the afternoon. This is usually not due to lack of nighttime sleep,

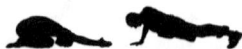

but is a function of a lack of physical activity for long hours during the day. This can also be magnified by low blood sugar from more than three hours without a healthy snack or from a lack of hydration. Most afternoon drowsiness can be cured by a walk, a drink of water, and a piece of fruit. The caffeine and sugar that most people depend upon are passive substitutes for the more active and healthy behaviors that are lacking from their daily routine.

A University of California, San Diego psychiatry study of more than one million adults found that people who live the longest report sleeping for six to seven hours each night. Other studies have shown that sleeping more than seven or eight hours per night is linked to increased mortality. Researchers at the University of Warwick and University College London have found that a lack of sleep can more than double the risk of death from cardiovascular disease, but that too much sleep can also be associated with a doubling of the risk of death, though not primarily from cardiovascular disease.

Professor Francesco Cappuccio has said that, "Short sleep has been shown to be a risk factor for weight gain, hypertension, and Type 2 diabetes, sometimes leading to mortality; but in contrast to the short-sleep/mortality association, it appears that no potential mechanisms by which long sleep could be associated with increased mortality have yet been investigated. Some candidate causes for this include depression, low socioeconomic status, and cancer-related fatigue. In terms of prevention, our findings indicate that consistently sleep-

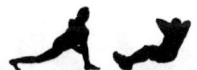

ing around seven hours per night is optimal for health, and a sustained reduction may predispose to ill health."

We all know that we feel terrible when we miss too much sleep and that over-sleeping makes us feel sluggish. Scientists have demonstrated that a lack of sleep can shorten your life. It contributes to increased occurrence of heart disease, obesity, stroke, and cancer. Several of these stem from the lack of opportunity for the body and mind to release the stress and exhaustion that accumulate during a typical day. Without sufficient sleep, the exhaustion and depletion accumulate and you literally wear your body out. I do not recommend a life like Rumpelstiltskin in which you sleep all of the time. But you need to let your body recover from a tough day by sleeping six to eight hours a night.

Four important keys to sliding off into a restful sleep are well known:

1. Establish a regular bedtime every night.
2. Stop using the computer at least one hour before bedtime.
3. Practice yoga or other form of relaxation as part of your fitness routine.
4. Stop using caffeine at least 2 hours before bedtime.

All of these will improve the quality and the quantity of sleep that you are able to get within an ordinary day. After telling you to exercise every day, you should be relieved to be able to balance that with a good night's sleep and short rest breaks during the day.

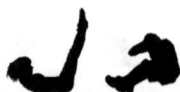

WEEKLY SHOPPING LIST

✔ *Just take a nap*

MUD 6.
RECHARGE THE HUMMER

Mud running will place additional demands on your body for nutritious foods and additional rest. The Blueprint recommendations for resting include getting eight hours of sleep each night, taking refreshment breaks throughout the day, and finding opportunities to release the mind to enjoy the beauty of nature.

Mud runners can add deep breathing and flexibility exercises during daily breaks. Stretch your muscles and fill your lungs to release stress and take in energy from your surroundings.

You may also take a few minutes to visualize the mud running course and prepare your strategy for each obstacle. If you have not previously run on the course you will be facing, then mentally rehearse past obstacles or watch video clips of the race to see what lies ahead of you. YouTube® mud running videos are great motivators. They show hundreds of normal people conquering the same obstacles you will face. They also show how some of the most seasoned competitors tackle these obstacles, so you can learn the tricks of the trade.

Visualization can help you get your mind into the zone for a mud run. It can release anxiety that you may have about competing in a new event. During the week prior to the race, watch its video several times for motivation and to get a picture of how you will handle it. Then incorporate those images into your rest breaks during the day.

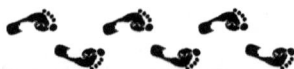

Week 7.
Six Meals a Day

What does "Three square meals a day" mean?

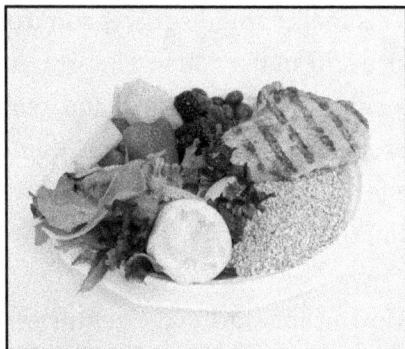

It has been the basis of healthy eating for generations. Mothers have worried that their children were not eating well if they did not have these "three square meals". We have all become programmed to include a daily time for Breakfast, Lunch, and Dinner. In our deep subconscious minds we believe that if we skip one of these daily milestones, then we are in danger of malnourishment or other health problems.

But where did this advice about nutrition come from? Was it a scientific breakthrough of the 1950's or as far back as the 1800's?

The idea is actually much older than most science. It dates back to the High Middle Ages around 1200 AD when knights still dressed in armor and attacked castles on horseback. For those who could afford to eat, food was served on a square wooden cutting board. If you were rich enough, then you had the money to eat three complete meals on these boards every day. So those who had three square meals escaped the effects of starvation and all of the diseases which took advantage of a weakened body. Three squares was the best defense against starvation, disease, and death over 800 years ago.

This makes three-squares some of the oldest nutritional advice still in use today. Unfortunately, this advice came from a time when starvation and real malnutrition were major problems. People were not watching their calories to shed a few pounds; they were watching their calories wondering whether they could get enough to survive another day.

Moving forward eight centuries, most of us now live in a time and place of abundance. Our biggest problem today is that our square meals are too big. We still use these "three squares" to fend off starvation, but now we measure starvation by the grumbling in our stomachs that occurs after 4 hours without food, rather than after 4 days.

Three square meals is an extreme example of the old, outdated technology of nutrition and fitness that many people are still following. In the centuries since the Middle Ages we have learned a lot about eating, but have not released our hold on those "three squares". Scientists now know that eating three times a day is a major contributor to obesity. Human blood sugar levels drop significantly two to four hours after a meal. As a result, people on the three squares plan arrive at each meal feeling famished because their blood sugar level is low.

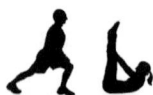

Their body chemistry is screaming at them to eat, Eat, EAT! So they follow orders and stuff food into their mouths until they just can't hold any more.

This overeating three times a day is making everyone fat.

Our outdated three squares habit is driving our body chemistry crazy.

Three square meals a day is a great way to avoid starvation. But it is a terrible way to remain healthy and fit. You have to reprogram and reschedule yourself for a new pattern of eating.

Your body will accept all of the food you eat, convert some of it into blood sugar, and burn that blood sugar in 2 to 4 hours. The rest will get stored as fat. At the end of four hours your blood sugar will be depleted and your body will send signals to your brain for a refill, preferably a BIG refill.

Most people follow a stuff-and-starve schedule like this

7:00 am	Breakfast
	Wait 5 Hours
12:00 pm	Lunch
	Wait 6 Hours
6:00 pm	Dinner
	Wait 5 Hours
11:00 pm	Sleep
	Wait 8 Hours
Repeat	

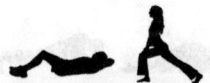

This puts 5 hours between Breakfast and Lunch.

It puts 6 hours between Lunch and Dinner.

And most importantly, it puts 12 to 13 hours between dinner and the next day's breakfast.

If your blood sugar is nearly depleted in 4 hours, that means that you have EAT, EAT, EAT signals in your brain at every one of the three square meals. These chemical signals are much stronger than your personal will power. The signals will force you to eat too much. The signals are making you fat.

So how do you get rid of the signals?

Do you diet and eat less? No. That will have the opposite effect.

You have to eat more often. You have to give our body healthy, nutritious fuel every 2 to 3 hours during the day. If you do this, then you will be in control of your urges, your choices, and the volume of food that you eat at each "meal".

You have to put the "three squares" nutritional advice from the Middle Ages in the trash and take on a modern 21st century solution to health. Six meals a day is not a "nice idea", it is an essential pattern for good health, weight loss, and physical development.

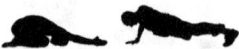

SIX ROUND MEALS

The new six meals a day are very different from the old three square meals. They are not a board filled with meat, vegetables, potatoes, gravy, and desert.

Instead, they are "round meals". Some are very small, others are a bit larger. Each one contains lean protein, complex carbs, healthy fats, fiber, and vitamins.

These meals are designed to give you nutrition throughout the day and to replenish your blood sugar before it is empty. The protein, fiber, and complex carbs will also fill your stomach and fend off hunger better than any junk food can.

Government Food Pyramid

Fats, Oils & Sweets
Use Sparingly

Meat, Poulyty, Fish, Dry
Beans, Eggs & Nuts Group
2-3 Servings

Milk, Yogurt & Cheese
2-3 Servings

Vegetable Group
3-5 Servings

Fruit Group
2-4 Servings

Bread, Cereal,
Rice & Pasta Group
6-11 Servings

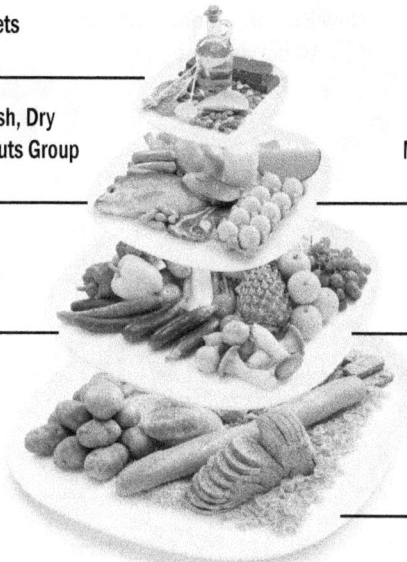

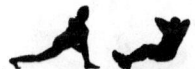

The government's latest eating guideline is a nutrition pyramid that identifies multiple servings of each type of food. This pyramid is heavily influenced by America's heritage in farming, with a large wheat and grain belt in the heartland. It prescribes far too many servings of bread and grains, even when those are healthy whole grains. If you add up all of the recommendations, the government plan calls for 15 to 26 servings of food a day. This would be at least 5 and as many as 9 servings in each of the three traditional daily meals. It is too much food.

We recommend a much leaner food pyramid based on vegetables, water, and lean protein. The New Blueprint Food Pyramid has a maximum of 15 servings of food per day, in place of the government's 26.

New Blueprint Food Pyramid
15 servings per day

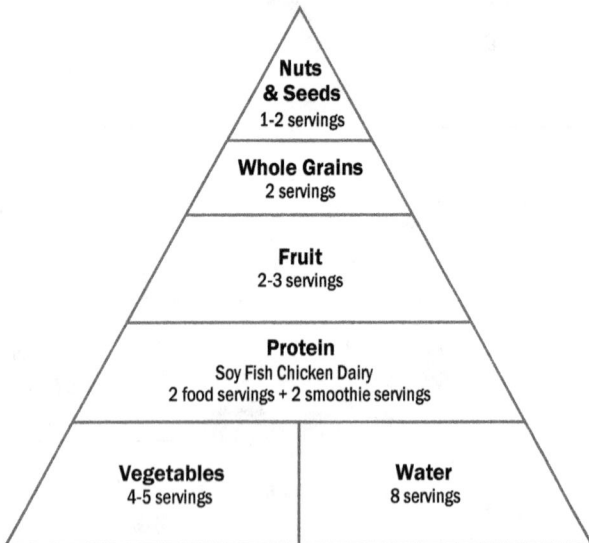

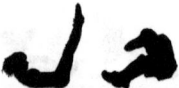

Nuts & Seeds
1-2 servings

Whole Grains
2 servings

Fruit
2-3 servings

Protein
Soy Fish Chicken Dairy
2 food servings + 2 smoothie servings

Vegetables
4-5 servings

Water
8 servings

If you are a professional athlete or intense physical laborer, then you probably need more food than this. But the average sedentary American should target 15 servings with between 2,000 and 3,000 calories per day depending upon your natural size. Since you will be eating nutritious raw fruits, fresh vegetables, skimmed milk, whole grains, and lean meat, you will be sufficiently fueled and filled in 15 servings rather than the government's 26.

You will also notice that the New Blueprint Food Pyramid does not contain a recommended number of servings of sugar. The recommended number is always zero. This pyramid is a model of what you should be eating. We will all splurge on sugars and fried foods occasionally, but we should not intentionally target a sugary desert in our diet every day by including it in the recommendations on the pyramid.

Tom says ...

— — —

"There are some great web sites for information and ideas on eating healthy. One of my favorites is *Self.com*, created by the same people who publish the *Self* magazine. They have one of the best nutrition databases on the regular foods that we eat. Also look at

- US Institute of Medicine's Food and Nutrition section: iom.edu/Global/Topics/Food-Nutrition.aspx
- USDA Choose My Plate: www.choosemyplate.gov"

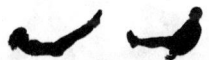

— — —

SCHEDULING SIX

What do six meals a day look like? How much do you eat at each meal and when do you have time for six of them? Here is one possible schedule.

7:00 am Breakfast	Protein Smoothie (see recipes in this book)
10:00 am 2nd Breakfast	Oatmeal with Raisins, Cinnamon, and Truvia®
12:00 pm Lunch	Chicken & Salad or Fish & Vegetables
3:00 pm Afternoon Snack	Nuts, Fruit, Diet Drink
6:00 pm Post Workout Snack	Protein Smoothie
7:00 pm Dinner	Chicken, Vegetables, & Beans

This schedule is just meant to give you a feel for the plan. You can work in your own choices for fruits, vegetables, oatmeal, protein, beans, fish, and chicken at the times that fit your taste and your working routine.

Many nutrition books provide long lists of good foods followed by more lists of cooking recipes. These are all great. But most people already know what is on those lists. They just choose not to create a daily meal plan that includes them. You know what foods are healthy. You just have to buy them, store them, and put them into your diet.

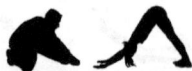

I decided not to include a list of foods in the New Blueprint for Fitness™. This is the framework for your new healthy lifestyle. You can fill in the details yourself from other food books and your own creativity.

FAST FOOD

Everyone eats out at "fast food" restaurants. This usually means someplace where you stand up to place your order and carry out your own trash. But there is little difference in the food at fast food restaurants and that at "sit down" restaurants. Both offer healthy and unhealthy choices. The people who make bad choices in fast food, also make similar bad choices in sit down restaurants. It is not so much the restaurant as the person who has a food problem. Two powerful cures for that are:

1. Eat six meals a day so you are not starving when you walk into a fast food restaurant. If your body chemistry is not screaming at you to EAT, then you will have much more control over the order you place when you are looking at the menu.

2. Choose to walk into a restaurant that has healthier choices on the menu. Skip the burger joint and pick someplace that focuses on salad, grilled chicken, or fresh burritos.

Tom says ...

— — —

"If the main dish at a restaurant is a burger and fries, then just don't go there. Keep driving until you find a place where the main dish is something healthier. There are many good food choices at those burger joints. But the question is whether you will choose those healthier meals. You are much more likely to eat healthy when all of the food on the menu is slanted toward the healthy side."

— — —

TWO MEALS IN ONE

When eating out you should almost always get a to-go box. Most meals served in restaurants are double sized. The sandwich, salad, or burrito that comes out of the kitchen will usually serve two normal people.

When your meal arrives, immediately cut everything in half. Put half in a to-go box. It will become a delicious meal tomorrow. This will cut your calories and put you on a path to some serious weight loss. It will also cut your eating expenses in half.

In the last few years a number of really delicious fast food burrito chains have opened across the country. Several of these focus on fresh vegetables and healthy meats. This is a great start. But most have made one serious health mistake.

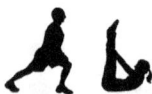

They prepare a burrito or a bowl that is the size of your head. It is too much food!

Do you remember the first time you visited one of these burrito places? You could barely finish half of the burrito that they gave you. But, over time, you expanded your stomach and your waistline until you could eat the whole thing. You need to return to the half-burrito serving. Always cut this soccer ball sized burrito in half. Save the rest for another day.

New Kind of Variety

Most athletes and fitness experts live on a very repetitive diet. They eat a small number of ingredients over and over again. Every breakfast is the same. They have two or three major choices for lunch and dinner. Their snacks are regimented. The variety comes from rotating the types of fruits and vegetables each day, not from entirely new dishes.

In a world of uncountable choices in food, the rest of us need to return to a more limited diet of healthy variety. You can sample new restaurants, new dishes, and new foods regularly, but the bulk of your daily food intake should be meals and snacks that you repeat over and over. These should be foods that are both very healthy and that you really enjoy eating.

Variety should be the spice of your life just once every few days, not at every meal. This week's shopping list provides a sample of the core foods that you should be repeating daily and which should be stocked in your kitchen.

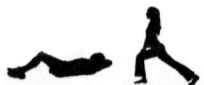

WEEKLY SHOPPING LIST

- ✔ Fresh Vegetables
- ✔ Fresh Fruit
- ✔ Chicken Breast
- ✔ Fish Fillets (no breading)
- ✔ Low Fat Milk
- ✔ Almond Milk
- ✔ Eggs
- ✔ Whole Grain Breads
- ✔ Quinoa
- ✔ Rice
- ✔ Plain Oatmeal
- ✔ Herbs and Spices

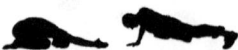

Mud 7. Grub Levels

Eating six meals a day will change the composition of your body. It will help you make good choices to eat more vegetables, fruits, whole grains, and lean proteins. Since you are not gorging yourself three times a day, your body will become more lean and muscular. It will morph into the ideal body type for mud running. Each pound of fat or even unnecessary muscle that melts away is one pound that you do not have to haul over a wall or carry on a four mile run. When people lose ten, twenty, or more pounds, they experience a lightening of their personal load. This weight is no longer pressing on their feet, pulling the spine out of shape, tasking their heart, or squeezing against their lungs.

Your mud run performance will improve noticeably when you lose a couple of pounds on a good six-meal diet.

Your body adapt to having fuel throughout the day. So it will be ready for action at any time, not just during one set daily exercise period.

PRE-RACE

Many people prepare for a big competition with a plate of spaghetti the night before. This practice began with the classic runners of the 1970's. It was not and is not based on the science of metabolism. It was just a hunch that seemed right at the time.

The meal from the night before cannot be completely digested and assimilated by your body for your morning performance. You should modify your diet for several days prior to a mud run.

Add an extra piece of fruit, a larger serving of lean protein, and some additional water. This little extra for three days will give you all of the energy you need for the race.

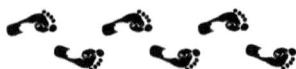

WEEK 8.
LEARN TO BURN

Trainers encourage people to "Feel the Burn." But most people are not really sure what that means. Exercise is hard work so they think that anything they are doing must be "the burn". In most cases, they have not reached it yet. Because they are not in the burn zone their workouts do not deliver the hard muscle, lean body results that they are looking for.

If you are not in the burn, then you will never get the kind of body that you see in the pictures. That level of fitness only comes from burning the fat, burning the muscles, and burning the lungs.

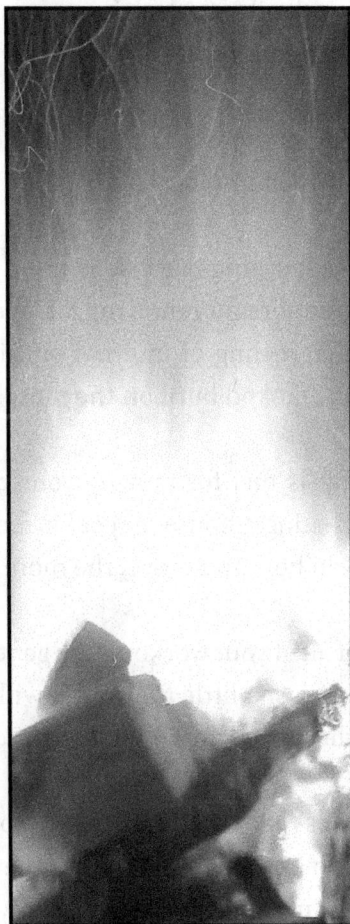

So what and where is the burn?

We use the word "burn" in fitness similar to its use in cooking and camping. When building a camp fire we pile on the wood, leaves, and fuel. Then we apply the spark that will ignite that fuel. The result is a roaring fire that creates a lot of heat, flames, and some smoke. This fire turns a big log into a small pile of ashes. It is an amazing transformation of matter into energy.

Exercise has a similar power to turn matter into energy—to turn fat into heat and action. But only if you do it right.

Fat burning exercise is not a gentle walk in the park. It is a campfire for removing fat. We talk about "the burn" because that feeling of internal burning is what it takes to burn off the fat and burn on the muscle.

Fat is fuel for moving your body, just like wood is fuel for heating a house, or coal is fuel for moving a train. The more you heat and move, the more fuel that is burned.

If all of your workouts are gentle and mild, then you are burning just a little fuel and it will take a long time to burn all of the fat you are trying to get rid of.

Most people have to "Learn to Burn". It is not something that comes to them naturally. They spend most of their time collecting and conserving energy—which is great when survival

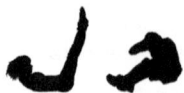

is at stake. But it leads to obesity in modern society where there is plenty of food and little danger.

Burn Like a Fire

For fire to turn wood into energy, a few basic ingredients have to be present. First, you need the fuel itself. Second, you need the spark to start the fire. Finally, you need oxygen to feed the flames.

Looking at the human body under exercise, it uses very similar ingredients. Most of us have plenty of fuel to burn. It is stored around our waist, in our thighs, packed to our behind, and hanging from the backs of our arms. Check—that one is covered. The spark for exercise is the motivation to get started and to keep moving. This book or exercise DVDs are great motivating sparks. Finally, the oxygen is in the air that you consume. Like a fire, a really good fat burn requires a lot of oxygen.

The more fuel you burn, the more heat you create. So a good measure of the amount of fat that is burning is the amount of oxygen you are sucking in and the amount of heat you are generating. You have to be doing enough work to cause heavy breathing and to raise your body temperature.

When you are working hard you generate a lot of internal heat. To get rid of that heat your body expels water in the form of sweat. This sweat releases internal heat and creates a thin radiator on your skin which will continue releasing ex-

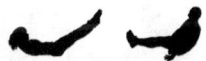

cess heat. So the amount of sweat coming out of your body is one measure of how much heat you are generating and how much fuel is being burned.

Your body has another mechanism for moving the oxygen around in your body so that it can fuel your muscles and trigger the fat burning process. That mechanism is the circulation of blood. Your blood cycles through your lungs, picks up oxygen, carries it out to the rest of the body, and returns carbon dioxide to be exhaled. When you are working hard your muscles need more oxygen and that can only be delivered if the blood is moving faster. So your body speeds up the blood pump—your heart. It beats faster and harder during exercise because it is trying to deliver more oxygen-filled blood to your muscles to fuel the burn.

Your heart rate, breath rate, and volume of sweat are all indications that your body is burning fuel. This fuel is the glucose stored in your muscles and the fat stored around your middle.

You cannot burn fat if your engine is not running hard. If your exercise routine is gentle and relaxing, you may be improving your flexibility or your balance, but you are not burning fat off of your body. Fat is a form of fuel and it requires real work to force it to burn.

The exercise DVDs that we recommended in an earlier chapter all provide great fat burning workouts. Stretching and gentle movement is a good way to warm-up for these work-

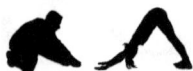

outs. But stretching alone will not burn fat. You have to fire up the engine, generate some heat, suck in the oxygen, and pump the blood around the body faster for fat burning to happen.

FAST AND SLOW

Wood burning fires are often described as fast burning or slow burning. A fast burning fire creates shooting flames and an intense heat. It can be so hot that you have to back up to avoid being roasted. This fast fire will consume wood in a much shorter time than will a slow fire.

A slow burning fire has glowing embers, almost no leaping flames, and a gentle radiant heat that you can stand close to for a long time. This fire puts out a much milder heat. It consumes the wood very slowly and can be kept alive all night long without completely consuming the wood.

Your workouts can be fast-burning or slow-burning. A fast workout with a lot of movement, sweat, and breathing will consume energy and fat very rapidly. You will burn the fuel in a much shorter time if you use a fast burning workout.

Fast burning workouts usually include movements like running, jumping, rapid calisthenics, and rapid weight lifting. Incorporating very short rest breaks between movements increases the intensity and the rate of the energy burn. Alternating exercises that focus on different muscle groups is a good way to reduce the rest needed between exercises,

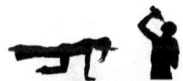

maximize the amount of work that you can do, and finish a workout in less time.

Tom says ...

— — —

"Your body is a machine for burning energy to perform work. Like a fire, the hotter it burns, the faster it consumes energy. This energy is linked to the glucose and fat stored in your body. So the most effective way to get rid of it is to dial up the heat of your workout."

— — —

A slow burning workout is something that you can maintain for a much longer period of time. You move gently, breathe much slower, and sweat little. This pace consumes energy slowly and you have to maintain it much longer to burn a significant amount of fuel. Slow burning workouts include walking, gentle bicycling, yoga, and Pilates.

Modern trainers design workouts that expend the most energy in the shortest amount of time. They recognize that most people cannot and will not consistently include a 60 minute workout in their day. So they have combined movements, sped up the pace, and cut out the rest breaks to put an hour's worth of exercise and fat burning into a 30 minute routine.

Many of the DVD training videos that we recommend offer this fast paced approach to fitness. This is not the only

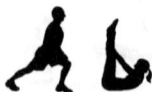

method that will work, but it is the one that best fits into most people's schedules and is exciting enough to continue for years.

There remain many benefits to a long, slow workout. But you must have the time and the calm temperament necessary to devote to these events. For a good workout, strive for the following:

- Move Fast
- Breathe Deeply
- Get that Heart Pumping
- Sweat Profusely

When you are doing all of these, you will know what the burn is first hand.

WEEKLY SHOPPING LIST

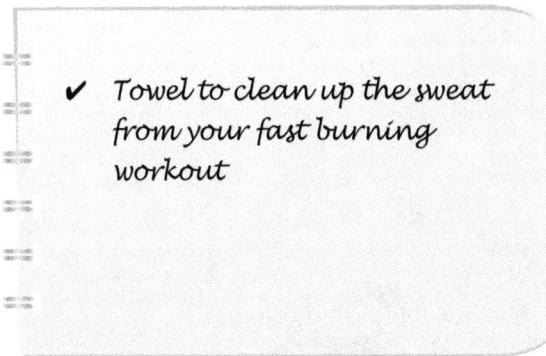

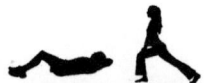

✔ Towel to clean up the sweat from your fast burning workout

Mud 8.
Burn With Hiit

What does "Burn" mean?

It is a workout which combines cardio and muscle build-ing together simultaneously, and during which there is very little rest. Weight lifters are notorious for working hard to get 8 to 10 reps of an exercise, and then resting for one or two minutes before the next set. That is not burning. They spend 75% of their gym time resting and 25% or less actually exercising. In a Burning workout you will do a dozen or more reps continuously for 20 to 45 seconds. Then you will rest for 10 to 15 seconds before the next set. You can also do one exercise for 30 second and then go immediately into a complimentary exercise without any rest at all. That is the burn.

Mud running is an intense physical workout combining cardio, strength, and flexibility. These challenges can come at you in quick combinations with little rest in between. Your training program needs to be designed to handle this kind of quick work load.

The high intensity interval training (HIIT) programs that are recommended in the Daily Exercise chapter will build a good mud running body. They will push you to keep working when your cardio and your muscles are tired. They will put you through a mini mud run every day.

These events attract people of all fitness levels. Many of them are the running athletes that you see training in the streets every day. These people usually have the cardio and leg conditioning to tackle the running sections easily, but they lack the core and upper body strength that they need for the obstacles. On every run I watch people take off ahead of me at a fast pace. But then I catch up to them and pass them on the obstacles. They struggle to use their upper body to get over a wall, rope ladder, or monkey bars. If they combined some HIIT workout with their running they would be much more outstanding in an event.

Workout every day and do not be afraid to get intense with it. Let a live or video trainer take you to challenging and uncomfortable places where you are tired, out of breath, and ready to drop. It will pay off when you are flying over an obstacle and leaving other people in the mud behind you.

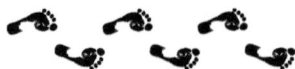

Week 9.
Hydrate

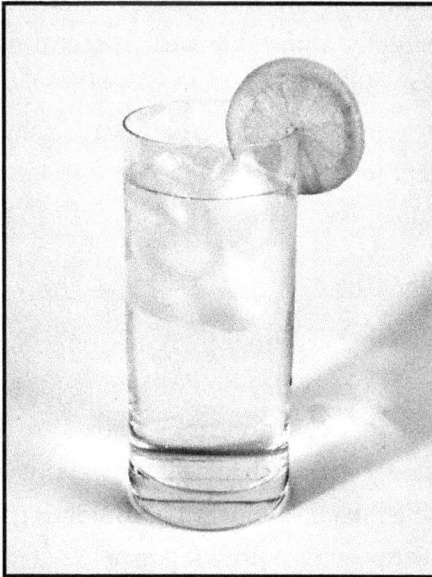

Water is the source of all life as we know it. This simple molecule of hydrogen and oxygen is essential to the basic function of life. When astronomers search the heavens for planets that can sustain life they look for signs of water. Scientists are not aware of any way for life to exist without water.

Over 70% of the Earth's surface is covered by water. If alien scientists were observing our planet from across the galaxy they would have no problem seeing that we are almost entirely covered in water. They would have to assume that there is abundant life on this planet.

Your body is similar to the planet Earth in that it is up to 60% water. It is actually a portable water processing plant that is constantly using and eliminating water as sweat, urine, and bowel movements. Small amounts are also lost through breathing, tears, and nasal fluids. Since this water processing plant is constantly losing water, it also needs to be coming in at a steady pace.

Most of us take this essential ingredient of life for granted. We run through a busy day only stopping for a drink when we really notice that our mouths or throats are dry, which is a biological signal that we have let our water levels drop too low. This is a big mistake. It is similar to starving yourself and then solving the problem with a big meal. That kind of eating will make you fat and out of shape. Depriving your body of water until it sends a strong signal has a similar effect. When that signal goes off, your body is already operating with too little water and some part of your body has already struggled with the effects of that.

When you become dehydrated your body slows down internal functions to conserve water and preserve life. This affects digestion, circulation, brain activity, energy levels, and

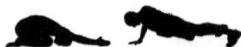

growth. To maintain and build a healthy body, you have to provide it with sufficient water throughout the day.

WATER FUNCTION

It is difficult to make a simple list of what water does for you since your body is mostly made up of water. The short answer is that it is involved in everything that happens in both your body and your brain.

Every fitness book contains a section on the importance of water. But my favorite is one written entirely about water. *Water for Health, for Healing, for Life* by Dr. Batmanghelidj carries the bold tagline, "You're Not Sick, You're Thirsty!" That is a fantastic statement about the importance of water in healthy living. Many of the aches, pains, and physical ailments that you suffer can be tied directly to having too little water in your body every day. Simply bumping up the number of glasses, bottles, or cups of water that you drink will make many of these problems disappear.

In his *Water* book, Dr. Batmanghelidj provides a long list of the functions of water in your body. Some of the most pressing are:

1. Water is the bulk material that fills the empty spaces in the body.
2. Water is the vehicle of transport for the circulation of blood cells.

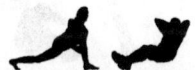

3. Water is the solvent for the materials that dissolve in the body, including oxygen.

4. Water is the adhesive that binds solid parts of the cell together.

5. The brain relies on water to move the sodium and potassium that are required for thinking.

6. Nerves require water to carry the electrical currents that signal movement.

7. Water stores and regulates the ingredients that create energy.

8. Water is the soup in which all chemical reactions take place to support the growth and repair of tissue.

Batmanghelidj's book actually provides many more vital functions of water. But these really got my attention when thinking about whether a little more water would do my body good.

WATER AND EMOTIONS

Through the centuries we have developed a pattern of believing that the mind and body are separate. We talk about emotions and feelings as entirely separate from the physical state of our body. This is completely incorrect. Emotions are created in the body by chemical reactions. They are a direct result of our physical actions, fitness, the foods we eat, and the water we drink.

This does not mean that all mental problems can be cured with food, water, and exercise. But it does mean that many

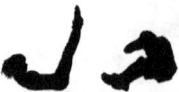

of the short-term moods that you experience can be significantly influenced by your physical habits.

When your body is short on water, this is often expressed through physical changes that you experience as changes in your emotions. These emotions can be moved in a positive direction with positive physical activity. Dr. Batmanghelidj has identified several emotional states that are influenced negatively by dehydration and positively by rehydration.

1. Tired without a plausible reason.
2. Irritable and unreasonably short tempered.
3. Anxious.
4. Dejected and inadequate.
5. Depressed.
6. Heavy-headed or slow to understand what is happening.
7. Disturbed sleep.
8. Unreasonable impatience.
9. Very short attention span.
10. Unexplained shortness of breath.
11. Cravings for coffee, tea, and sodas.
12. Night dreams about oceans, rivers, lakes, and pools.

This is a very bold list of claims. If you struggle with one or more of these chronic issues, then you should put this theory to the test. All you have to do is drink more water every day for a week and watch for emotional changes.

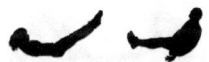

WEIGHT LOSS

Fitness books and trainers also tout the importance of water in a weight loss program. This simple ingredient has no calories and is very effective in curbing unhealthy habits and encouraging healthy ones in their place. Water ...

1. Is healthy to consume in large amounts.
2. Contains no calories.
3. Promotes the complete digestion of food and the absorption of nutrients.
4. Speeds digestion, moving food out of your bowels.
5. Fills your stomach and reduces the feeling of hunger.
6. Helps you lose weight by replacing the space of food in your stomach.

Drinking water is like eating food. You need to have a regular supply throughout the day. Do not wait until you feel thirsty or dehydrated before your start drinking. For weight loss, do not wait until you feel hungry to drink a glass of water to stave off hunger. By then it is too late. Your body will not be fooled by water with no calories. It will continue to demand food. Instead, you need to drink water every hour. The constant supply will create a fullness in your stomach that will push away the desire to snack.

When this is combined with six healthy meals a day, it will put you in control of your diet in both volume and the type of food that you consume. Even eating six times a day, some people feel strong urges for sweet and salty snacks every

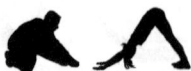

hour. Drinking water every hour is a good way to control those urges.

WATER PUNCH

Some people believe that "water" is a general term that includes tea, soda, coffee, alcohol, and sugary drinks. As a result, when counting their water intake they include all of these as well. That is wrong. Each of those drinks contains ingredients that the body uses pure water to digest. The benefits of the water contained in those beverages are used up by digesting the other ingredients that are in the drink. As a result, the water does not become available to the body for the essential core functions.

When I talk about drinking water I mean plain, old fashioned, clear, simple, refreshing water. It does not have a color, a flavor, or a caffeine boost. There is a place for all of those other drinks. But they are not a substitute for plain water.

Tom says ...

— — —

"Stop hating water. It is a delicious and refreshing drink all by itself. Drink it cold, warm, or at room temperature. Sip it slow or chug and entire glass in seconds. Start loving water again."

— — —

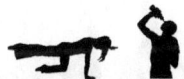

We all need to renew our healthy and simple relationship with water. We need to get used to drinking it plain without pouring in a powder, mixing it with flavors, carbonating it, or adding sugar. But, if you find that water is too boring to drink over and over all day long, there are a number of different water recipes that you can use to give it a taste boost.

1. Add ice to make it cold and more refreshing.
2. Heat it up like a tea and use it to warm you from the inside out.
3. Add a little sea salt to cut the taste of the chemicals.
4. Squeeze in a little lemon or lime to give it zest.
5. Add a little stevia to sweeten and overcome a mineral taste.

Adding lemon, sea salt, or stevia are not ideal. But these are much better than alternatives like drinking soda or drinking nothing at all.

WATER HABITS

Drinking water is a habit that you have to develop like any other. It is something that most people do not do enough of now and need to teach themselves to do more. You can do this by setting a goal for the day, making a plan to achieve it, and preparing the items that will make it possible. This is not a project like building the space shuttle. It is not climbing Mount Everest or swimming the English Channel. We are just trying to pour a little more water into your body. There is no cost barrier. There is no time barrier. There is very little

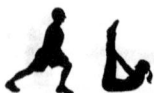

taste barrier. There is just a laziness barrier that has to be overcome.

Goal. Drink 64 ounces of water per day. That is 8 x 8 ounce glasses, 4 x 16 ounce glasses, or 2 big quart cups. It is best to spread this out through the day, so I would recommend using 8 to 16 ounce glasses or bottles.

Plan. Keep a glass or bottle of water with you all day long. Have one on your desk, carry one to meetings, and walk around the job with a water bottle. Empty and refill the bottle every two hours. So you should finish off a bottle of water in between each of your six meals a day. You can also include an 8 ounce glass with each meal and snack. That would easily take care of most of your daily supply.

Equipment. Get your own stylish and functional water bottle. Do not rely on sipping from a fountain. These sips are too small to add up to 64 ounces every day. Do not rely on pre-bottled water. If you are buying bottled water, both your wallet and your mind are going to try to skip the expense. It is much better to carry your own bottle and refill it at the many free sources that are in most homes and offices.

Your water bottle should be something that looks good and which works for your lifestyle. If you are going to have it with you, it needs to be something practical. Many people choose to refill some commercial water bottle like their last Dasani® or Sobe® bottle. Those bottles are very

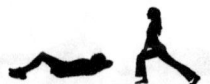

solid for reuse. If they become a little mildewy you can easily throw them in a recycle bin and start with a new one. They do not need to travel back and forth to the dish washer.

The bottled water craze is strong in America. So you can easily carry one of these around with you and everyone will see you as both healthy and progressive. There is no negative stigma to carrying water wherever you go.

WEEKLY SHOPPING LIST

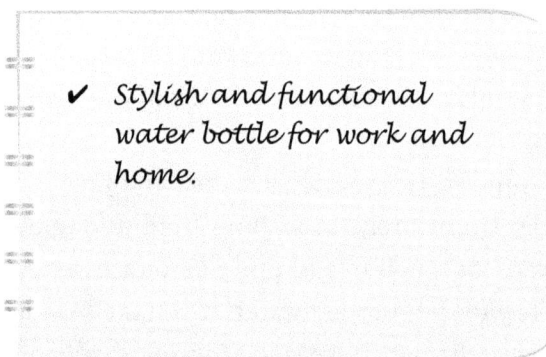

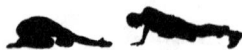

✔ Stylish and functional water bottle for work and home.

Mud 9.
Drink Up

During the two days before a race be sure that you are getting all of your fluids. The water you drink on Thursday and Friday will be fully infused into your muscles and organs when you are racing on Saturday.

Hydrate on the morning of the race as well—but nothing more than normal. The water you drink Saturday morning will be available for your muscles later in the race. But much of it will also rush to your bladder and send you to the port-a-potty when you are trying to get lined up for the race. You do not want to have an overwhelming need to relieve yourself when you are in the middle of the race trying to get up a wall.

You can also hydrate on race day with wet fruits like oranges, pears, and melons. The fiber in these will help to keep that water from heading to the bladder too soon.

A sports drink with electrolytes will also work for both pre and post workout hydration.

POST-RACE

Many of these races will hand you a beer as you cross the finish line. That is one source of fluid and carbs. But my favorite combination immediately after a race is:

- 12 ounce sports drink
- 8 ounce low fat chocolate milk
- 16 ounce water

I drink all three of these after the finish line and each never tasted so good. I can feel the hydration, electrolytes, and carbs refreshing my body as I take these in.

You should also have plenty of water in your car when attending a race. In most cases you will not need anything drastic. But just in case it is a very hot day or your body fluids are not balanced, you want to be able to hydrate as much as necessary. You will also be prepared for friends at the race who need an emergency dose of water.

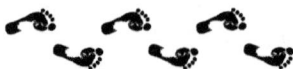

WEEK 10.
SMALL CHANGES

Everyone has some bad habits when it comes to nutrition, exercise, and rest. We all intend to be the best, fully committed, all in, guru of fitness—enjoying all of the benefits of good health. But when it comes time to put it into practice every day, day after day, there are some practices that we just cannot keep up with.

You have to accept some of this. Sometimes you have to do your best and let the rest take care of itself.

Building healthy habits is like building a bridge. It goes up over time. You have to lay a foundation to build up your strength and move on to bigger goals.

To keep getting better you have to experiment with new ideas and new practices. For those behaviors that are especially dif-

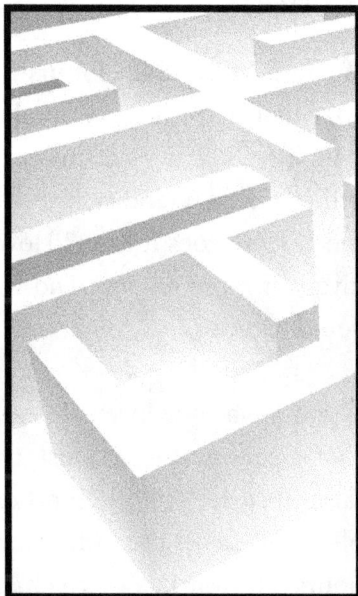

ficult, let yourself experiment with a newer, healthier choice just once or twice. You can get a feel for how hard it will be and also for the benefits you can expect.

Think about some of the improvements that you could make in eating, exercising, resting, and drinking water. Could you experiment with a change for just one day to see what it is like and how well it would work for you?

EATING

If you have trouble eliminating hamburgers and fries from your diet, then just try an alternative for one meal and see how it feels. The next time you are in a burger joint, order a grilled chicken sandwich and a salad. Give it a try for just one meal. How does it taste? How do you feel afterward? Did it give you more energy? Did it digest better? Did it improve your attitude?

If you are a soda lover, this afternoon when you are craving that sugar or caffeine boost, try something different. Try low fat milk, a zero calorie sport drink, or plain old water. Drink plentifully. Feel the difference. Notice what happens in the hours afterward. Is this a change that you could make more often?

If you have a candy bar regularly, next time reach for a piece of fruit. Try a banana, apple, orange, pear, peach, or blueberries. Would these be a better fuel for your body? Did you get a similarly satisfying energy boost from the fruit?

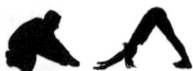

You like to snack on potato or corn chips every day. Give salted or unsalted nuts a try. They contain more protein, fiber, and healthy fats than chips. They will satisfy that need for something crunchy and salty. You will feel fuller and have more energy for a longer period with nuts than with chips.

You usually order fried fish for dinner. Just once ask for grilled or broiled fish. You will get more of the real fish flavor, less of the breading and much fewer calories.

You salt your food liberally. Try using herbs, lemon juice, pepper, jalapenos, or salsa to bring out the flavor in the food.

You use ketchup or mayonnaise on your sandwichs. Replace this will salsa and some extra vegetables. These add plenty of flavors and bring the same moistness that you get from ketchup. When ordering a sub sandwich I like to tell them to put on "all of the vegetables". They do not charge extra for this and it can double the size of the sandwich. It will even help you skip the chips.

EXERCISE

You find it difficult to do a workout every day. There is always something more important to do. For just one week, insist on a daily workout at a set time. Put it on your calendar and do not let anyone move it. Experience daily exercise for one full week to see if the benefits are worth the discipline it will take to maintain it.

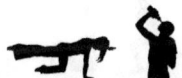

Getting up in the morning for a short metabolism boost is just too hard. You feel that you need that few extra minutes of sleep to get through your day. For one week, get up 15 to 30 minutes earlier and spend that time exercising. Go for a walk around the block or pop in a short workout DVD like the 10 Minute Trainer®, a short yoga or Pilates stretch, or Jackie Warner's 15 minute total body workout. Do this for seven days in a row and watch your energy that week. Did the exercise give you more energy than the sleep that you normally get?

If you usually take the elevator in your building, start by walking down on the stairs. You can still ride the elevator up to a higher floor, but go down using the stairs and invite those with you to do the same. Did this make a difference in your alertness and energy level during the day? If so, then try adding the up direction next week.

WATER

It is just too much trouble to be constantly filling and draining water bottles. For just a single day purchase four 16 or 20 ounce bottles of water. Drain two of them before lunch and two after. Do you feel any different? Can you tolerate the few extra trips to the restroom?

When you practice this, buy water in bottles that are nice enough to refill in the future. Few people can maintain a habit of buying four bottles of water every day.

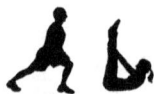

New Habits

These are just a few of the most common habits that are difficult to build. You can use this trick with any new habit that you are trying to acquire. Give the newer, better behavior a full day or a full week to get the best feel for what you can expect. Then do it again in a few days or weeks.

Our lives are built on habits. These are patterns of behavior that we have become comfortable with. They solve practical problems in our day by eliminating long decision-making processes and replacing those with automatic behaviors. We go through every day partially on auto-pilot. This is a good thing because it allows us to save our mental and physical energy for the unique events of the day—those that require creative new solutions.

But it is also a bad thing because we believe that we cannot change these old habits. We become so connected to them that we will not allow ourselves to release them. Changing an old habit always leads to changes in your mental and physical state. It requires spending a little extra time thinking about what we are doing. But once the new behavior is repeated a few times, it becomes the new programmed habit.

Habits are a common self-preservation behavior that has protected humans for eons. But they are also a set of behaviors that hold back progress, change, improvement, and goal achievement. You need to be regularly upgrading your hab-

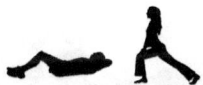

its. Once you have mastered the past and present, you create new habits that will move you into the future.

Keeping the same habits for years will just cement you to the past. In the area of fitness, it will insure that you are in exactly the same shape a year from now that you are in today, which is exactly where you were the year before that. Becoming healthier, stronger, and happier require creating new habits that will replace the old ones.

Getting fit is not like having a surgical operation. A surgeon can fix what is wrong with you in a few hours. When he is finished, the problem will be gone and you can get on with your life in your newly repaired body. Fitness relies on a set of habits that will be part of your life for years to come. You are changing the way you live, not just for a month, but for the rest of your life.

Let yourself develop new habits. Swap out old behaviors for new and better ones.

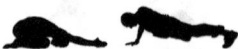

SOME SWAP IDEAS

Old	New
Hamburger	Chicken
French Fries	Salad
Soda	Water
Candy	Fruit
Chips	Nuts
Fried	Grilled
Salt	Pepper
Mayonnaise	Salsa
Work All Day	Workout Every Day
Sleep Late	Morning Metabolism Boost
Sipping Water	Guzzling Water
add your own below	

Mud 10.
Fuel Fit Fun

Mud running calls for a few basic, but consistent changes to your lifestyle. Luckily most of these are fun and enjoyable.

Fuel Daily. Every day you need to give your body good fuel to work with. You should take in two or three servings of vegetables and fruits daily. Feed yourself complex carbohydrates like oatmeal before your body chemistry forces you to substitute those for sugar. Finally, get good servings of lean protein from fish, chicken, milk, eggs, soy, and powders. These will turn your hard work into a performance body instead of a couch body.

Fit Daily. Your body is made to perform physical work every single day. The rest you get from sleep and the energy from food are made to move the body and the mind. Your exercise routines can vary from one day to the next, but there is no reason to have a day with no physical activity at all.

Fun Daily. It is unfortunate, but most people need to be told to do something fun every day. Society pushes so many "must do" and "need to" activities into our lives that we begin to believe that the purpose of every moment is to work on some problem. We deny ourselves the joy of doing things that really bring us happiness and pleasure. Or we push all of our fun into a single day of the week. That is wrong. Everyone should be having at least one thrilling, happy, enjoyable activity every day. This is not decadence; it is owning your life.

Thrill Weekly. If you are having fun every day, then the mud run is the thrill of the week. Once you are in physical shape for it, a mud run can become something that you look forward to every single weekend. It can become like your father's weekly game of golf. On Friday evening golfers will get their gear together, make sure the car is full of gas, check the fridge for the necessary beverages, then go to bed in eager anticipation. For the new fit generation, we go through these same ritual preparations, but when we arrive at the golf course we jump into the lakes and climb the trees instead of hitting the little white ball.

Team Connection. Mud running creates a very tight social bond with other maniacs who are willing to crawl through a mud hole. Look for social groups in your area, join a team, or create a team. These bring encouragement and excitement to every event. They will also help you keep track of the races in your area, organize road trips, and be there to help out if you run into problems.

Try one of the largest mud run teams in the country, Mud Run Fun—http://www.mudrunfun.com/.

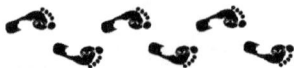

Week 11 through 1100. Just Keep Going

This book contains a lot of great advice and guidance on becoming fit and living a healthy life to 100 years old. But all of this writing, talking, and thinking is worth nothing if you do nothing.

If you have reached this chapter according to plan, then you have spent a week focusing on each of the ten core habits in your new blueprint for fitness. That is a great achievement and one worthy of celebrating. You have already gone further than most people who make a New Year's resolution.

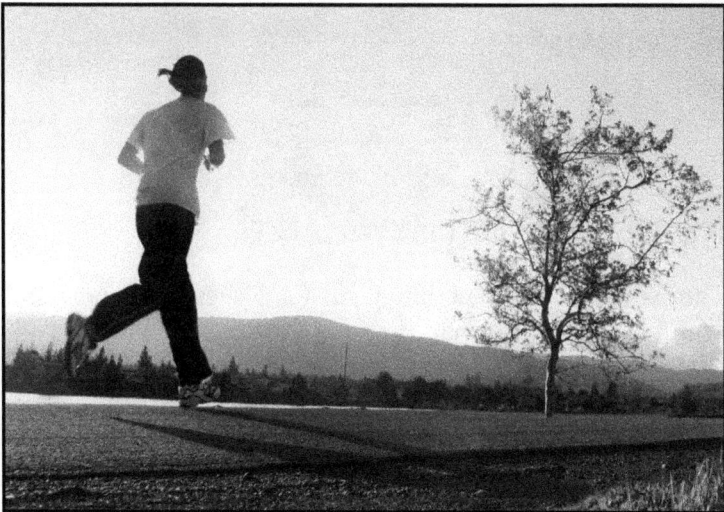

But you are not at the end. You are at the beginning.

You followed the advice for weeks one through ten. The advice for weeks 11 through 1100 is to just keep going.

You have seen changes in your own body.

You can feel the difference when you wake up every morning.

These changes are just the beginning. It gets better every week that you keep going. The 1100 weeks ahead of you are not a grind, they are a joy that grows continuously. If you keep going you will be physically, emotionally, and spiritually enriched for the rest of your life.

Tom says ...

— — —

"Just keep going."

— — —

New Blueprint, New Habits

The habits of the New Blueprint for Fitness™ support and build on each other. The additional rest that you incorporate into your days and nights will work together with your morning metabolism boost to give you more energy all day long. This energy is further supported by a healthy breakfast, smaller meals, and your healthy snacks throughout the day.

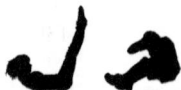

These will give you more than enough energy for your daily workouts and every other activity of your daily life. This blueprint is captured in a single graphic that will remind you of your new goals and behaviors. There are also several copies of this blueprint at the end of the book. Cut some of these pages out and post them where you will see them every day. Share them with the people who comment on your new look and your new habits.

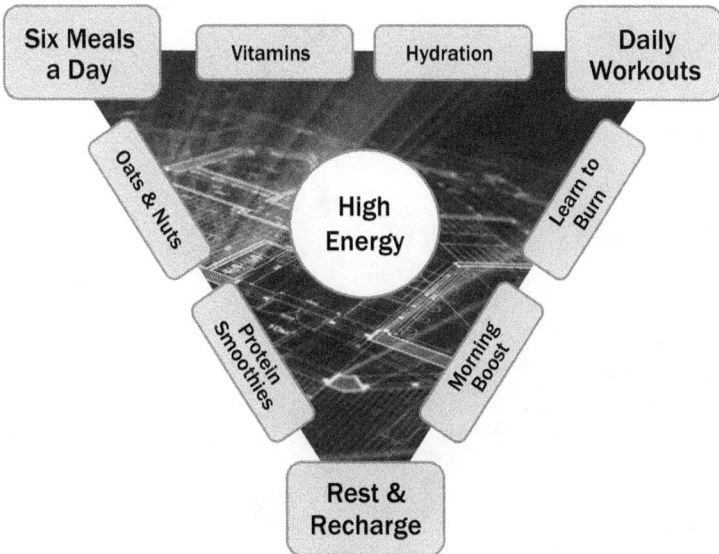

Welcome to a new set of habits and behaviors that make up the New Blueprint for Fitness™ for the rest of your life.

Just Keep Going.

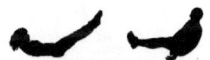

Mud 11 Through 1100: Muddier

Once you get into shape for life, sports, and mud runs, you are on the path to a new lifestyle. This is not a quick fix, it is a permanent change. From now on your lifestyle will include healthy eating, exercise, regular rest ... and for you mud runners, a regular weekend romp through the mud.

Each event is different in the same way that each golf course is different. After a half dozen you will begin to detect your own personal strengths and weaknesses on the course. Like athletes in other sports, you will enjoy and capitalize on your strengths, but you will also work on improving your weaknesses. Like a golfer who can drive the ball a thousand yards, but cannot putt even a few feet, you will tweak your body, skills, and performance to get better at those especially tough obstacles.

All mud runs are not targeted at the same audience. Some are meant for the casual weekend participant, others for regular athletes, and a few for the most hard core competitors. As you talk to other people and jump into a few events you will discover these levels and create a path through them for yourself. You may want to have a relaxed fun experience every time. Or you may be looking for a hard core challenge, attending the easy ones only as training sessions for the really difficult runs.

Just keep going.

This is a very new, young, and growing phenomenon. It is a bit too wild and unruly to be called a sport yet, but a structured competitive sport will emerge and become part of the X Games® in the future. For now, enjoy the challenges and the chaos.

There are going to be a number of spin-off events from mud running. It is so creative and unbounded that it will generate specializations and unique new twists. If you are participating regularly, watch for these twists and give each a try. Right now no one knows where this is going to go, but it is going to be a fun ride.

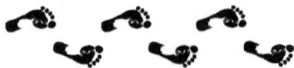

MOTIVATION
& TIPS

OWN YOUR LIFE

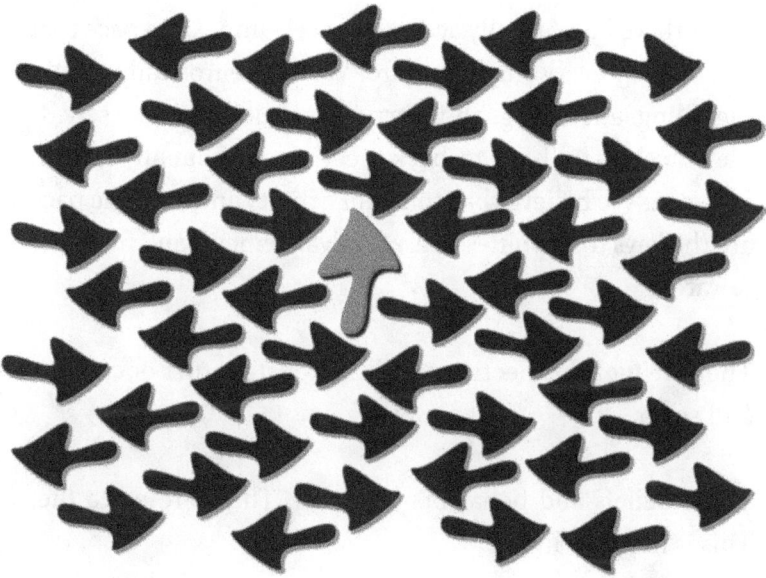

The most common argument against a healthy lifestyle is, "I don't have the time." People believe that they do not have time for a workout. They cannot afford to take a 10 minute break in the morning and afternoon. They have to rush through lunch. They cannot get to the grocery store to buy healthy foods for the house. There is no free time in the afternoon for a workout.

But what are we all so busy doing? Are we always working to put food on the table and pay the bills? Or are we watching television, surfing the internet, checking our social networks, and playing video games?

The truth is usually that we have plenty of time to make our own choices.

At work we have usually accepted or self-imposed a pace that has us busy every single minute. We are neurotically checking, filing, answering, and worrying about email. We schedule ourselves for back-to-back meetings without any time in between. We believe that constant activity and a frantic pace are the keys to happiness, career advancement, and financial reward.

Then we fuel this hectic day with a constant diet of caffeine and sugar.

These beliefs and behaviors are crazy. These are not a life. This is not fully living.

Regardless of what your boss implies, you are the owner and programmer of your own life. You can and do choose what you will do every day. Unfortunately, many people have chosen to work 24/7 and reserve no piece of the day for themselves. Is that the path that you are following now? Is that the path that you want to follow? It is a fast and furious path to the grave. You are racing to the grave without spending any time on the things that are important to you.

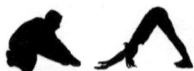

Is that the life you want to choose for yourself?

Is your greatest dream to be available 100% to your boss, your social network, and your television schedule?

Do you have any other dreams?

Most of us wish we did not have to give all of our time, energy, and attention to the things that are important to other people. We wish that we could preserve some of that for our own dreams, our own moments of satisfaction. We wish ... but we do nothing.

To build a fit body and a healthy lifestyle, you are going to have to stand up and take back a few minutes of YOUR day. The time and energy that you have all belong to you. You may have chosen to give all of it to someone or something else. Now you are going to choose to take some of it back for your own fitness and health.

Welcome to ownership, control, and responsibility for your own life ... all of it. Stop living someone else's dreams, schedules, and deadlines. Start investing in yourself. That is how you are going to have the time that you need for a new healthy lifestyle.

THE SQUEEZE

When all of the ideas in this book are taken separately they sound like they will eat up a huge portion of your day. You imagine that you will be doing nothing all day but servicing your new healthy habits. But many of these behaviors can be combined into a short 5-10 minute routine, killing three birds with one healthy stone.

By combining everything, you add only about 60 or 90 minutes to your day. This is about half the time that most people spend watching television each day. Only 45 minutes of this is your daily workout and the rest slips into the middle of your day in short 5 to 15 minute pieces. Here is one example of packing all of these new behaviors together.

20 Minute Morning Jumpstart

2 Glasses of Water
Metabolism Boost—Walk Outside or 10 Minute Video
Protein Smoothie—Lots of Ingredients
Vitamin Pill

15 Minute Mid-Morning Break

2 Glasses of Water
Oatmeal Packet with Cinnamon, Raisins, and Truvia®
Walk Around the Office
Step Outside for Fresh Air and Sunshine

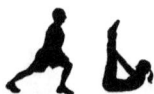

Healthy Lunch

2 Glasses of Water

Turkey and Salad

Diet Soda or Tea (if necessary)

10 Minute Mid-Afternoon Break

2 Glasses of Water

Fruit & Nuts or Protein Bar

Stretch at Your Desk

45 Minute Workout

Vigorous Exercise

Post-workout Protein Drink

1 Additional Glass of Water

Healthy Dinner

Fish, Salad, Fruit

Whole Grain Bread

Stop

No food 2-3 hours before bed.

No caffeine 2 hours before bed.

No water 1 hour before bed.

When you take control of your life you will find time in YOUR day for the things that are important to YOU. 60 to 90 minutes is not impossible, it is your own personal claim on the energy and time that all belong to you.

Your Muddy Life

Your first few mud runs can be intimidating. If you
have not been to one before, it can be a challenge
to complete the registration process. Your mind is filled
with images of young, super fit models conquering impossible obstacles. That is a distorted picture of the
entire experience. Mud runs attract people of all ages,
sizes, and fitness levels. Most of us are far too ugly to
appear in the promo videos. They turn the camera away
when we come into view. But we are all there.

At a big run there will be hundreds of people who are
the same age, fitness level, and appearance as you. You
will not be unusual looking. In fact, in this crazy sport
it is almost impossible to look weirder than the people
who attend regularly in wild costumes. Relax, everyone
is struggling just like you are.

Here are a few tips for getting started.

Muddy Step 1. Register. So don't postpone or weasel out
of the first step. Put your fears behind you and throw
yourself in, you will have a great time. If you register a

few weeks early you will have more choices of starting times and lower prices.

Muddy Step 2. Map. These events are not held in your local city park. They require lots of raw open land. So they are off the beaten path. In most cases you will not have been anywhere near these locations. That means there is the real possibility that you will get lost driving to one. Print out a map to the site or load it into your GPS. Don't let a wrong turn rob you of the fun.

Muddy Step 3. Show Up. When Mud Run Saturday Morning arrives it is easy to open one eye and say ... I'm too tired ... the weather is too cold ... it rained last night ... I am sore from a workout ... I need to mow the grass. Do not entertain any of these thoughts. You already decided that you were going to show up when you registered. Today you just follow through with that great decision.

Get out of bed, dress in your gear, and pack the car. Once you are at the site and surrounded by other crazy people, the shared energy will erase your excuses and make you eager to get started.

Muddy Confession: One morning I woke up for a mud run, stepped outside and decided that it was too cold to be jumping into a muddy pool of water. So I dressed and spent the day doing responsible chores around the house. Within a few hours the temperature was up and it was a beautiful day to be out in nature. But it was too

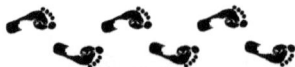

late to make it to the run. I spent the entire day regret-
ting that decision and decided that I would never listen
to my morning excuses again. If it truly is too cold to
get wet, then I will just skip the water obstacles. But
that is a decision that I can make when I am standing
on the course, not when I am crawling out of bed.

Muddy Step 4. Live Your Full Life. Too many of us have
accepted or created a life in which we act responsibly
all day every day. We no longer let ourselves play. Use
this new hobby to give yourself permission to have a
thrill. Live a life that you would be interested in hear-
ing other people talk about. That can start with a small
weekend mud run. The thrill can become infectious,
spurring you to actually have fun every day of the week.
Mowing the grass or shopping for groceries should not
be the most exciting part of your weekend.

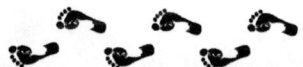

Tips & Tricks for Your Personal Blueprint

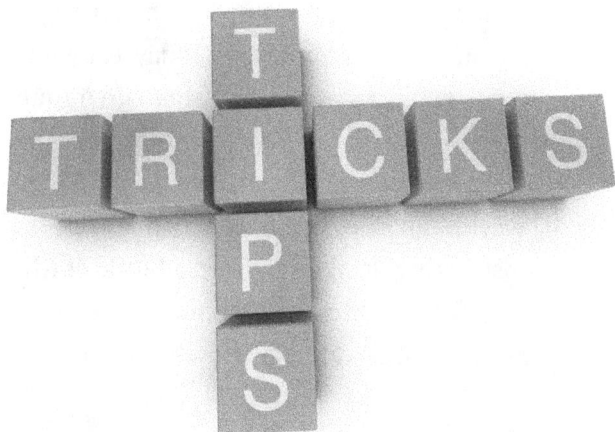

People who have worked on their fitness for years have discovered a number of very useful tips for getting the most out of the time, energy, and money that they invest. Fitness magazines and books are filled with these tricks. Some of those that have helped me in the past are shared here to get you started.

Morning Metabolism Determination. Do not decide whether you are going to walk or exercise when your alarm goes off. You have already decided that you ARE doing it. So, get out of bed, take your bio break, and drink two glasses of water. Then put on your casual clothes and step outside. Now you can decide. Breathe the air. Listen to the birds. Feel the temperature. Now make the decision about being part of the world today.

Energy Shortage. If you are too tired to do a workout in the afternoon, it is a good sign that you are not eating a healthy snack one to two hours before your workout. If you had eaten fruit, a protein smoothie, nuts, or a protein bar, then your energy would be fine. Fix this tomorrow. Today, eat your snack now and you will feel like a workout in about 30 minutes.

Water Bored. There are times when water tastes like the best thing in the world. But once you have satisfied your thirst, it can be the most boring drink ever. Keep a bottle of Mio® flavor drops handy. Squirt a little into a bottle of water to really jazz it up. Don't skip your water, give it a flavor boost.

Choke on a Pill. If you are one of those people who are too squeamish to swallow a vitamin pill, then try a different brand. Some great options are: (1) the smallest pill you can find, (2) chewable, or (3) gummy vitamins. The worst vitamin is the one you will not take. All of these choices are better than that decision.

No DVD. If you are still living in the Stone Age without a DVD player, then you will have to use your computer for the exercise routines. What, no computer either? Then you are going to have to follow the exercise pictures in a book. The books by Jackie Warner and Tony Horton are both excellent.

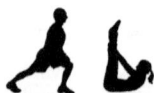

Running and Jumping. If you are significantly overweight and/or just getting started in fitness, then you should avoid running and jumping. Both of these activities put a lot of stress on your feet and joints. If those are not ready for it, then you are going to end your fitness career in a hurry. There is plenty of time to add these exercises in six months or a year. Just wait.

Shoes. What kind of shoes do you need for fitness? Some people believe that the most expensive shoes make a difference in their performance and the health of their feet. But others believe that feet have evolved to walk, jump, and run best when barefooted. It appears that most foot problems like planar fasciitis started with the invention of the modern running shoe. Maybe you foot muscles, like the rest of your body, need to be free to exercise when you walk. You do not have special gloves to help you with computers or musical instruments. So why do you need special shoes to help you walk? I do my workouts in a thin pair of "toe shoes" and find that this has improved the strength of my feet.

Back Pain. The more whole-body, dynamic exercises that you use, the less trouble that you will have with your back. Core, Yoga, and Pilates routines make a noticeable difference in relieving back pain. If you are using many of the modern training programs that incorporate these exercises you will reduce and perhaps eliminate the pain in your back.

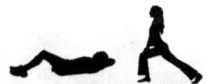

FOOD CHOICES

Everyone in fitness will tell you that a good diet begins in the grocery store, not in the kitchen. When you load your grocery cart you are deciding what you will put into your stomach. If it comes home with you, you will eat it. If it does not come home with you, there is no way for you to get at it. So do your shopping after you have had a healthy meal and look for the foods that you know need to be in your diet every day.

Real Food. We have gotten so far from our farming roots that we have forgotten the difference between real foods and manufactured foods. The shelves of the grocery store are filled with foods that have been manufactured for taste, convenience, and profits. Real foods are those that contain exactly one ingredient and were taken directly from nature in the form that you pickup in the store. These include raw fruits and vegetables, plain meats, nuts, seeds, milk, and eggs. Closely related to these are the combinations of ingredients that are only one step removed from nature, such as oatmeal, yogurt, cheese, whole breads, and juices. Everything else has been manufactured to appeal to consumer tastes, shelf life, and corporate profit margins. Your diet needs to include big servings of real foods and those that are just one step removed. In this modern age, none of us are going to eliminate all of the manufactured foods. But eat those after you have had a good helping of real foods.

Fruits are real food which means that they will actually spoil. You should always have fruit in the house, but in limited

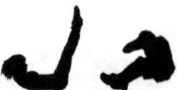

amounts. Stock only as much as you can eat in one week. Beyond that you risk losing it to rot.

Vegetables with Dressing. Salads are an important part of your daily diet. You can spice these up in a number of ways. The best is to add vegetables, fruits, and nuts with tastes that you really like. These could include carrots, apples, orange slices, radishes, bell peppers, pecans, walnuts, or almond slivers. The second is to add a low fat salad dressing. Something based on olive oil and vinegar is great and it avoids the fats that come in the creamy varieties. My favorite for all kinds foods is Ken's Steak House® Lite Caesar. I use a small amount of this on salad, fish, chicken, and anything else that is too dry or too dull to enjoy alone.

Whole Grain Bread. Bread is supposed to be brown and heavy. It is made from wheat and other grains that are brown and heavy. The only way to make light, fluffy, white bread is to tear the wheat apart and take out everything that makes it nutritious. All that is left is enough starch (carbs) to make the bread stick together.

Smoothie Ingredients. The key to making delicious and interesting smoothies every day is to have the ingredients in the house. You must have the protein powder, fruit, plain yogurt, almond milk, 100% juice, ground flax seed, and cinnamon in the house to be able to satisfy your thirst for this liquid power.

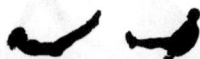

Low Fat Milk. Opinions are mixed on the value of milk. I believe that it is a powerful nutrient similar to nuts -- both contain the power of new life and growth. If you are lactose intolerant you are going to have to use a lactose-free brand. But, I believe that everyone else should include low fat milk in their diet every day.

Museli Cereal. It is difficult to find a manufactured cereal that can really be recommended as a healthy choice. Look for muesli that does not have added sugar or whole wheat biscuits that are the same. You can eat these in small quantities for breakfast. I prefer to pour them into a coffee cup to control the portion size. A typical cereal bowl is actually 2 or 3 servings, not just one.

Nuts. These are the seeds of new plant life on earth. You need to include these powerful foods in your diet and have them for regular snacks.

Chia and Hemp Seeds. Native tribes have used these as a primary food source for centuries. They have fueled some of the longest surviving and fastest running civilizations in history. Give these a try in your protein smoothie to feel what they can do for you.

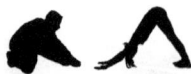

MUDDY TIPS & TRICKS

There are a number of tips that will make you a better mud runner. But, don't get hung up on every detail. You will do just fine without any prior planning or preparation. Thousands of people jump in every weekend and have a great time without worrying about it.

Tip #1: Signup, show up, have a good time, and don't get hurt. If you are doing these, then you are 90% of the way there. The rest is gravy.

Tied Tight. At my very first mud run I asked the pro who was expected to win the race for one piece of advice he would give to a newbie. His advice was, "Tie your shoes tight. The mud will suck them right off if you don't". So I am passing that to you as well.

Dry Materials. Cotton is a wonderful material for clothing ... when it is dry. But when wet it is heavy, soggy, and holds water a long time. Your race is going to take you through mud, lakes, rivers, and bogs. You do not need to be carrying five pounds of water with you in your shirt, shorts, socks, and underwear. Choose a synthetic material that lets water drain off quickly. These products have a dozen different names, but they are usually made from a synthetic material like rayon, perhaps with some cotton included.

Running Hydration. Throughout the race there will be water stations where you can get a few ounces of fluids. In the thrill of the moment many people do not feel thirsty and do not notice that they have perspired significantly, so they bypass the water stations. Mistake. Always grab a cup and have a little water at these stations. Trust your plan, not your feeling of thirst.

Wet Off. At the end of the race you will be covered in wet clothes. When your body temperature is up, these can feel very comfortable. But they are also wicking away your body heat much faster than normal. Within 20 minutes of finishing the race you should change to dry clothes. Do it before you start to shiver.

Dress Fun. Mud runs are athletic parties; wild dress-up costumes are always welcome. You can wear absolutely anything you like. From roman gladiators to ballet dancers and superheroes, everything goes. Be comfortable, have fun.

Team Up. Look for a team to join, or create your own team. It could be a group that runs together for the fun and energy, or it could be a competitive group. These teams will help you show up, perform better, and have

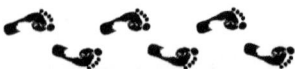

more fun. Try Mud Run Fun (http://www.mudrunfun.
com/) as a starting place.

Carb Up. If breakfast is the most important meal of
the day, then the breakfast before your mud run is 10X
more important. Do not go into an event with an empty stomach and low blood sugar. Have a sticky bowl of
oatmeal and a protein drink the morning before the
race.

First Aid. Each race will bring its minor scrapes and
cuts. Keep some disinfectant and bandages in the car.
When you are cleaning up after the race, clean and
bandage your wounds as well. So far I have never gotten
an infection from a cut on my leg that was then repeatedly dipped into mud, lake water, and tree branches.
Maybe it's the vitamins and daily exercise.

Drug Store. Newbies will often pop an ibuprophen or
other pain killer right before or after a race. It keeps
away some of the soreness from the stressed muscles
and bruises you will pick up on the course.

Personal Shower. Races sometimes provide a primitive
outdoor shower at the finish line. Sometimes they just
point you to a pond or lake where you can jump in to
get "clean". If you want to insure a basic cleanliness at
the end of the race, bring two gallons of water with you.
You can be your own shower station in the parking lot.

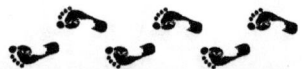

Gloves. I have a pair of rubber gloves in my race bag, they are "Pugs" purchased at 7-11 for $4.99. I have carried these with me on a couple of runs, but never actually used them. But other people wear gloves for every race.

Leggings. Compression sleeves that come up to your knees are very popular. The most common scrapes are on the shins and calves. These socks can significantly reduce cuts from the underbrush and wooden obstacles.

Photo Op. You can carry your own waterproof camera on a lanyard or in a pocket. Novice competitors are not shooting for record breaking time, so there are plenty of opportunities to stop and take pictures of yourself, friends, and the course. Many races hire professional photographers to get pictures of the racers. You can purchase or download these from the web in the days after the race.

Beach Towels. When the race is over, you have had your shower, and you are ready to get out of your wet clothes, you may find no private place to change clothes. Experienced runners come prepared to do the beach change. They wrap a towel around their waist (men) or entire torso (women) and use it as a private changing booth. Slide the wet clothes off and the dry clothes on inside the towel.

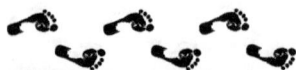

Sun Block. Since these runs usually occur in the spring and summer, you will want to put sun block on your exposed areas. Certainly cover your head, face, and neck. Most people spend at least an hour on a short course, some as long as three hours. So this is significant exposure that calls for some protection.

Lip Balm. Protect your lips in the same way you protect your skin.

Optional Obstacles. Mud runs are a fun, casual, personal challenge. This is not the NFL. You can tackle the course anyway you like. Every obstacle is optional. If you come to an obstacle that is too hard for you or that triggers an inner phobia, you are free to skip it. These courses are laid out to challenge people at every level. There are always a few obstacles that are meant only for the experienced, super-fit competitors. Leave those for the pros. If there are 30 obstacles on the course and you skip 2 or 3, then be proud of the 27 or 28 that you conquered and forget the rest. As you become more experienced you will conquer the tough ones as well.

Run vs. Walk. The events are called mud runs, but walking in an option as well. If you cannot run the entire 5 kilometers, 10 kilometers, or 10 miles, then feel free to walk along the way. You will find that many of the casual competitors are doing the same. One Saturday I signed up for two different mud runs that were just 40

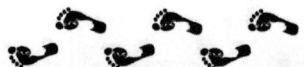

miles apart. I gave my all at the first one. But when I arrived at the second my knee was too sore to run, but it felt fine when walking. So I walked the entire course. I had just as good a time in slow motion as I did running. And I still beat a number of people because of my fast performance on the obstacles.

Fun. You are out here to have fun, so do not forget to do that first.

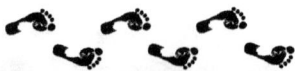

BLUEPRINTS TO GO

We have included several copies of the fitness blue-print for you to cut out and post in your home and office. These will remind you to stick to your new habits for fitness and health.

You can also share these with friends who notice the changes in your own body and lifestyle and want to know how you are doing it.

THE NEW BLUEPRINT FOR FITNESS™

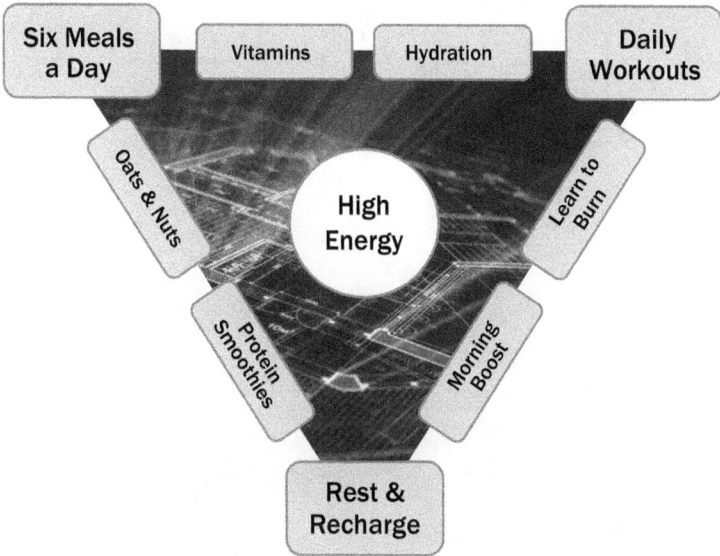

Six Meals a Day — Vitamins — Hydration — **Daily Workouts**

Oats & Nuts

High Energy

Learn to Burn

Protein Smoothies

Morning Boost

Rest & Recharge

www.NewBlueFit.com

THE NEW BLUEPRINT FOR FITNESS™

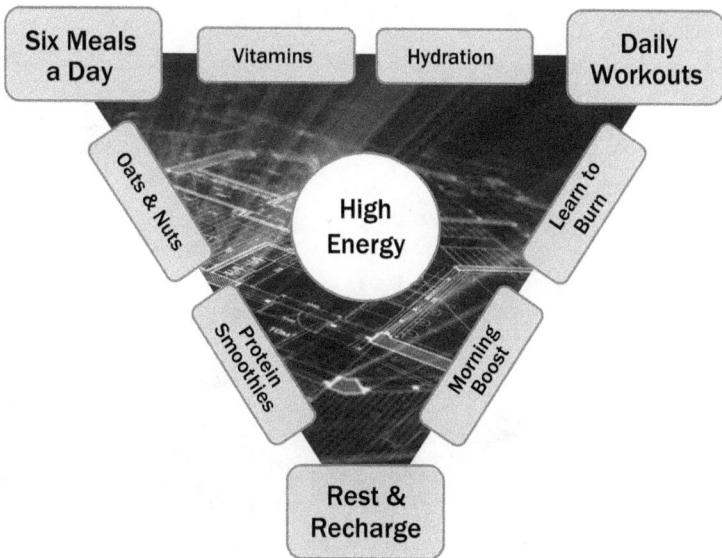

Six Meals a Day

Vitamins

Hydration

Daily Workouts

Oats & Nuts

High Energy

Learn to Burn

Protein Smoothies

Morning Boost

Rest & Recharge

www.NewBlueFit.com

THE NEW BLUEPRINT FOR FITNESS™

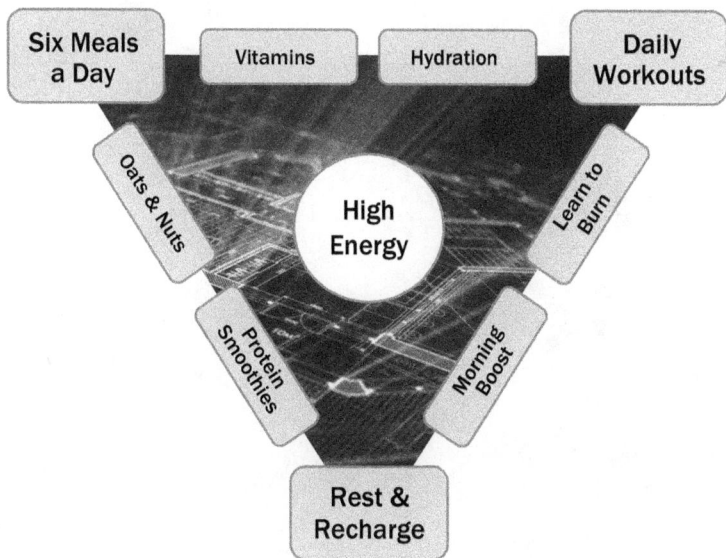

Six Meals a Day

Vitamins

Hydration

Daily Workouts

Oats & Nuts

High Energy

Learn to Burn

Protein Smoothies

Morning Boost

Rest & Recharge

www.NewBlueFit.com

THE NEW BLUEPRINT FOR FITNESS™

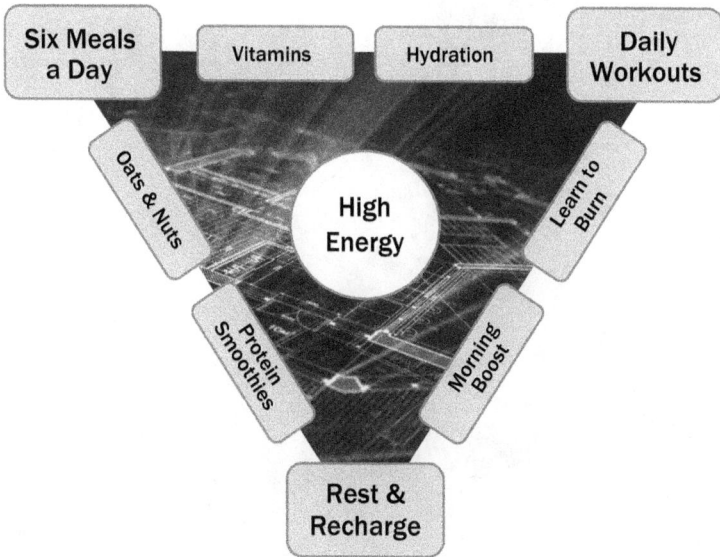

Six Meals a Day · Vitamins · Hydration · **Daily Workouts**

Oats & Nuts · **High Energy** · Learn to Burn

Protein Smoothies · Morning Boost

Rest & Recharge

www.NewBlueFit.com

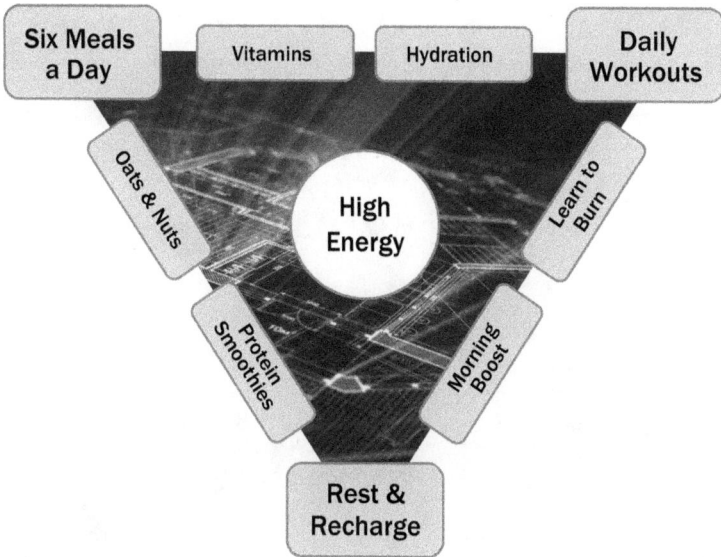

Six Meals a Day

Vitamins

Hydration

Daily Workouts

Oats & Nuts

High Energy

Learn to Burn

Protein Smoothies

Morning Boost

Rest & Recharge

www.NewBlueFit.com

THE NEW BLUEPRINT FOR FITNESS™

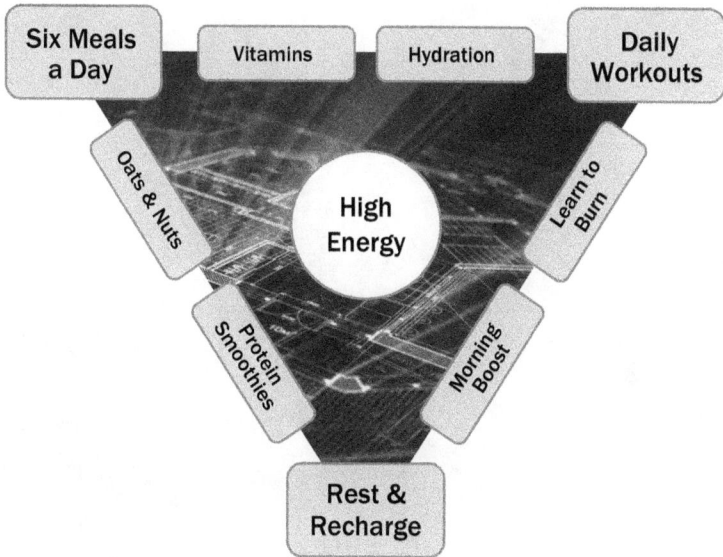

Six Meals a Day | Vitamins | Hydration | **Daily Workouts**

Oats & Nuts

High Energy

Learn to Burn

Protein Smoothies

Morning Boost

Rest & Recharge

www.NewBlueFit.com